T0127086

the Happy Body

Praise For

The Happy Body

"Coach Jonathan Wong has compiled an informative manual that bucks the conventional "knowledge" on nutrition and exercise, and raises the bar on fitness. This book connects the dots between the emotional challenges of forging your own path in eating well and strength training, and provides you with the guidance you need to help you reach your health goals."

—**Esther Blum**,MS,RD,CDN,CNS,
Best Selling Author of *Eat, Drink & Be Gorgeous*
http://www.livinggorgeous.com

"I consider *The Happy Body* to be an incredibly useful owner's manual for anyone who has a body and who wants to know how to move, feed, and heal their body for optimal functioning."

—**Kim Frazier**, Masters in Integrative Medicine, Duke University

"*The Happy Body* attacks all the aspects of fat lost issues. From the relation of fat loss and hormonal issues, quality and quantity of food, even the relation with the people that surrounds you, type of training to use, everything is covered! Most of all, Jonathan uses his own experience with countless satisfied clients, to give all the tools for the reader to reach his goal!"

—**Christian Maurice**, Celebrity Fitness Coach, Montreal, Canada
http://www.christianmaurice.com

"As a fitness coach for over ten years, and an avid reader and researcher or information in the health and fitness industry, I found

The Happy Body to be a very usable and comprehensive guide to optimal health. I will certainly be recommending it to my clients and family."

—**Glenn Stewart**, Strength & Conditioning Coach, New Zealand

"Working as a therapist and a performance trainer, I'm getting to see a lot of people each day. I will definitely recommend this book to my clients, friends and family. This book will help them to achieve their goals and answer their questions in the best way possible. If you want to change your life in to the better, and achieve optimal health, this book is for you. This book will in an easy way help you to make the right choices and answer your questions about a getting the healthy body you want.

This is a great recourse and a must in your bookshelf."

—**Einar Svindland**, Dr. of Naturopathy, Norway

"Jonathan Wong is a friend and fellow Coach who has shared much the same mentors as myself. He has distilled the gems from all these experts and in this book boils it into a caring simplicity of not overdoing anything or looking at components of the body "through a straw". It is a journey into optimizing all that is good without falling into the trap of thinking more is better. The way the auto fanatic knows their owner's manual inside and out, Jonathan has given those dedicated to holistic health that same manual but for the human condition. This book belongs on everyone's shelf."

—**Mike Demeter**, Senior Nutrition Consultant,
Goodlife Gyms Canada

"*The Happy Body* takes a complex topic and makes it simple for even laymen to understand. It's packed with practical suggestions on how to achieve your health goals, and an essential tool for anyone looking to change his life for the better."

—**Daniel Chong**, Economic Analyst

As a life-long competitive sportswoman, I found *The Happy Body* to be packed full of advice that has been useful to me both on and off the field. The information on sleep, treating pain and strengthening was especially beneficial for me. I would heartily recommend it to sports people that are keen to improve their performance.

Coach Jonathan Wong has applied his many years of training and experience to this book. It is clear that he is serious about helping people achieve their ideal "Happy Body"."

—**Lesley Sim**, National Frisbee Team, Singapore

"*The Happy Body* encapsulates the essential principles required for everyone to lead a healthier and a more holistic lifestyle. I used to be overweight and tried many methods to lose weight, only with limited success. I also had poor sleep quality and low energy levels. *The Happy Body* addresses how to overcome all these issues in the wide range of topics that are covered in this book. Over the past year, I've applied these principles and the results have been great! I am no longer overweight, I enjoy better sleep and I am embracing the higher energy that I now have. Most importantly, I am grateful that *The Happy Body* has changed my previously myopic perspective on how I view health and fitness."

—**Charmaine Su**, Lawyer

"*The Happy Body* is a great one-stop reference tool for achieving long lasting health and performance in all aspects of life. The ideas in the book have helped me greatly in attaining my fitness goals as an athlete, and continue to guide my everyday decisions with regards to maintaining an optimum state of well being. The injury treatments Jonathan has used on me and other athletes to address some chronic pain issues and have proven to be safe and very effective. A must for every bookshelf!"

—**Jesper Chong**, National Floorball Team, Singapore

"The ideas on nutrition, supplementation and exercise that I learned from *The Happy Body* really helped me get my weight and blood sugar issues under control. I used to be on medication for blood pressure and diabetes, but after just a few months, my medical doctor has cleared me to get off all medication."

—**Jason Chen**, IT Systems Analyst

"Taking the integrated, step by step suggestions in *The Happy Body* allowed me to overcome many of the health issues I was facing. Previously I had poor sleep, bad digestion and terrible energy levels, especially when I woke up in the morning. These were all addressed by the topics in the book."

—**Jessica Fernandez**, PhD Candidate in Material Science

"I have recommended this book to my colleagues and family members because it is very focused on helping people make changes which can show benefits pretty quickly. Following the detoxification plan really helped me a lot with energy levels and weight issues because my former occupation as a safety inspector for oil tankers exposed me to high levels of petrochemical toxins."

—**Charles Yen**, Safety Inspector

"I had been struggling with chronic back pain since the birth of my second child. Following the exercises and stretches recommended in *The Happy Body*, along with dry needling treatments as suggested in the book for my kind of pain, I am now pain free and can continue chasing my kids around the way a young mother should."

—**Christy Leedon**, Mother of Three

H*the*appy Body

Getting to the Root of
YOUR *Fitness, Health*
and *Productivity*

JONATHAN WONG

NEW YORK

the Happy Body

Getting to the Root of YOUR *Fitness, Health* and *Productivity*

© 2013 JONATHAN WONG. All rights reserved.

No part of this publication may be reproduced or transmitted in any form or by any means, mechanical or electronic, including photocopying and recording, or by any information storage and retrieval system, without permission in writing from author or publisher (except by a reviewer, who may quote brief passages and/or show brief video clips in a review).

Disclaimer: The Publisher and the Author make no representations or warranties with respect to the accuracy or completeness of the contents of this work and specifically disclaim all warranties, including without limitation warranties of fitness for a particular purpose. No warranty may be created or extended by sales or promotional materials. The advice and strategies contained herein may not be suitable for every situation. This work is sold with the understanding that the Publisher is not engaged in rendering legal, accounting, or other professional services. If professional assistance is required, the services of a competent professional person should be sought. Neither the Publisher nor the Author shall be liable for damages arising herefrom. The fact that an organization or website is referred to in this work as a citation and/or a potential source of further information does not mean that the Author or the Publisher endorses the information the organization or website may provide or recommendations it may make. Further, readers should be aware that internet websites listed in this work may have changed or disappeared between when this work was written and when it is read. The material in this book is for information purposes only. Each person is unique so you should use common sense, in partnership with a qualified healthcare practitioner before using the methods and information in this book. The author and publisher expressly disclaim responsibility for any adverse effects that may result from the use or application of the information contained in this book.

ISBN 978-1-61448-427-1 paperback
ISBN 978-1-61448-428-8 eBook
Library of Congress Control Number: 2012935392

Morgan James Publishing
The Entrepreneurial Publisher
5 Penn Plaza, 23rd Floor
New York City, New York 10001
(212) 655-5470 office • (516) 908-4496 fax
www.MorganJamesPublishing.com

Cover Design by:
Rachel Lopez
www.r2cdesign.com

Interior Design by:
Bonnie Bushman
bonnie@caboodlegraphics.com

In an effort to support local communities, raise awareness and funds, Morgan James Publishing donates a percentage of all book sales for the life of each book to Habitat for Humanity Peninsula and Greater Williamsburg.

Get involved today, visit
www.MorganJamesBuilds.com.

Dedicated To

God, our Creator, who made us in His image. The magnificent precision and beauty by which every aspect of our being operates all demonstrate His fingerprints of loving design.

I will praise thee; for I am fearfully and wonderfully made: marvelous are thy works; and that my soul knoweth right well.
—Psalm 139:13-15 KJV

TABLE OF CONTENTS

FOREWORD

Overall, the health of our society is deteriorating. The rates of cancer, heart disease, diabetes and obesity continue to rise. Who is responsible for this health crisis? The government? The pharmaceutical industry? Fast food? New viruses? Antibiotic resistant bacteria? The cost-cutting approach of managed health care? No! We are all responsible for our own health. The level of health that we enjoy today is a direct result of the decisions that we made yesterday. And the choices we make today will affect our well-being tomorrow.

Jonathan Wong's Happy Body teaches us how to make these healthy choices using both time tested and cutting edge strategies. This light, practical, effective and entertaining guide succinctly covers all of the major aspects of health and healthy living. You can read it cover to cover (which I highly recommend) or each chapter is complete and cross referenced so that you can effectively target your area of concern (like sleep or weight loss). Whether you are a novice or an accomplished health care provider, the happy body has something for everyone. As Jonathan says "Getting old is guaranteed but aging is optional."

Wishing a "Happy Body" to all!

—**Robert A. Rakowski**, DC, CCN, DACBN, DIBAK
Clinic Director, The Natural Medicine Center, Houston, TX

ACKNOWLEDGEMENTS

Here is a list of people who, by their teaching, their work or their support have made this book possible.

- my loving and supportive wife Priscilla, who has allowed me to disappear for hours into the study room to write;
- my parents Doreen and Kok Leong who have taught me the character traits that helped me push this book through completion;
- my siblings, who have given me perspective and inspiration during the process of writing;
- my fellow coaching team at Genesis Gym Singapore, who have taken such great care of our clients while I was taking time off to write; and
- every single client who has passed through our training center in the last eight years of our fitness center's existence. It is our team's journey and experience in learning how to help you that gives me the confidence to write this book with conviction and certainty.

My mentors, who have shared their years of experiences, and given me the knowledge to help a wide variety of clients with their health goals:

- Olympic Coach Charles Poliquin and his education team at the Poliquin Strength Institute, which conducts probably the finest strength training education program in the world;
- Dr. Rob Rakowski for his expert guidance in nutrition and disease prevention. And I am equally grateful to him for writing the forward to this book.
- Dr. Allan Austin and Dr. Mark Scappiticci who have, by their experiences with Olympic teams, and through their mentorship and courses, shown me what world class injury prevention and rehabilitation looks and feels like;
- Dr. Mark Houston whose seminars, videos and books on cardiovascular health have helped give me the confidence to care for this group of at-risk clients.
- Dr. Johnny Bowden whose practical approach to nutrition has helped me make consistent healthy changes in the lives of others;
- Dr. Mark Schauss whose dedicated work in laboratory testing and detoxification has helped me get results with even the most difficult client cases; and
- all of the other teachers, professors and healthcare practitioners who have dedicated their lives to the well-being of their patients and students and whose books and other educational material have helped my team and I give consistently good outcomes to the clients under our care.

INTRODUCTION

I'm a "teach a man to fish" kind of guy.

In fact, about 90% of the clients I have helped over the last twelve years don't want to see me anymore! While some may argue that this is "bad for business," to me, this is a great success. Allow me to explain…

In my practice as a health professional, my objective is to lead client on a journey to discover the real reasons behind their health problems. Once they know the source of a problem, they can use the strategies suggested to keep that problem away for good! So, they may not need my services as often as before.

I'm a big believer in education and in people taking responsibility for their own health. In fact, my team and I at Genesis Gym spend a great deal of time educating clients. As a coach, I am responsible to each client and patient, trying to provide each of them with the best possible information and advice.

The meaning of *health*, *fitness* or *energy* can be different for each person. A competitive athlete may consider a more explosive vertical jump as better fitness. While, for a busy female executive, great looking arms in a sleeveless dress may be a more important fitness goal. Someone more senior may consider fitness the ability to live independently and enjoy a high quality of life as he or she ages.

No matter what your definition of health is, there are fundamental processes and systems in your body that need to be taken care of to achieve maximum results. These systems are covered in this book.

Before you feel discouraged and think that this is going to be a biology or anatomy textbook, rest assured, it is not. *The Happy Body* is a book that covers subjects in enough detail to help you understand why it's a good idea to treat your body well, without confusing or boring you with biochemical reactions or anatomy charts.

Most importantly, the key aspect that sets this book apart from other health related books is that you will learn how all of these systems in your body interact to help … or hinder you in achieving your health and fitness goals

While I may not have a doctorate in any particular subject of health, I've become very adept at searching out the best in fields of health ranging from exercise, to nutrition, to rehabilitation and management of chronic diseases so that I can receive coaching and mentoring from them and in turn, provide the best information to my clients for all of their health and fitness goals.

The information in this book is compiled from more than sixty seminars, certifications, conferences and internships, hundreds of hours of travel, and thousands of hours of study and practice. I then apply this knowledge to the hundreds of clients my team and I serve each month at the two facilities that Genesis Gym operates in Singapore.

This pool of knowledge is updated continually as I learn more. Only methods, products and systems that have worked for me, my clients and my colleagues in the field of holistic health are included.

Very importantly, the solutions presented make sense from a proper understanding of how our bodies work in general, yet also from an understanding of how different we can be as individuals.

For example, we should all eat most of our food from unprocessed sources (general). However, the amount of starchy carbohydrates that we should eat varies from person to person according to things such as our genetics, activity level and current level of body fat (individual).

How this book is structured

Because your body is one integrated being, it is important to know how the parts work together for optimal function and maximum health. There is no start or end to how your body is put together; this book is arranged in such a way that front to back reading may not be as effective as using the book as a reference guide to seek out the information that's right for your unique individual needs.

What I suggest is for you to start with the chapter that best describes your current health condition. For example, if you have constipation, start with the chapter on digestion. Each topic is a short explanation about the causes of each problem, and what methods are effective in dealing with the problem.

More importantly, within each topic are directions to other sections in this book that explain related areas for you to read, which can help you find root causes of your problem and even more solutions.

Because of these many inter-chapter links, there may be some overlap in the symptoms, causes, and solutions in the topics covered in *The Happy Body*. I will do my best to avoid repeating myself, and if a related topic is covered in greater depth somewhere else in the book, I will point you to the right section and page to find out more about it.

Links Between Related Topics

These links are in brackets and underlined bold font. For example, a link to Chapter 2 section 2.3.1 would look like "**(2.3.1)**". In fact, if you dig deep enough you will see, through the linkages from topic to topic, how incredibly your body works, and how improving one area, can help you maximize your health in many others. I believe the knowledge that you have such an awesome piece of machinery in your care can be a powerful motivation to improve your lifestyle, habits and health. Treat this book as a strategic map for your journey to more complete health and wellness.

Please enjoy the ride.

PS: On the companion website to this book, there are videos to explain things that are learned better by watching rather than reading. Go to www.happybodybook.com to see the videos that can help you understand the information in the book more clearly.

Chapter 1

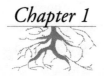

Some Basics

No matter what topic you are starting with, some basic things hold true of how our bodies work. Be aware of these ideas as you read the other chapters.

1.0 Your body gives you clues

Your body is an incredible piece of machinery that can give you feedback to help you find out which areas you may need to look at to maximize your health. Here are some common problems you might be facing, and what problems they could indicate. You can then turn to the sections of this book that can help you best.

Problem: Poor energy levels

Possible causes:

- stress hormone imbalances,

- poor nutrient levels, or
- poor sleep quality/quantity.

For possible solutions, check chapters 3, 4, 6 and 9.

Problem: Poor recovery from exercise

Possible causes are:
- lowered muscle building hormones,
- poor sleep quality/quantity, or
- poor nutrient levels and digestion.

For possible solutions, check chapters 3, 4 and 9.

Problem: Poor mood and motivation

Possible causes are:
- a brain chemical imbalances,
- poor nutrition, or
- sleep and stress-related issues.

For possible solutions, check chapters 6 and 9.

Problem: Health-related issues for women (e.g., irregular menses, tender breasts, premenstrual syndrome).

Possible causes are:
- imbalances in female hormones, or
- excessive stress levels, (which also interfere with hormones).

For possible solutions, check chapters 9, 10 and 11.

Problem: Hunger and cravings

Possible causes are:
- poor blood sugar management

- non-optimal brain chemical function
- stress related eating

For possible solutions, check chapters 4, 6, and 9

Problem: Digestive issues

Possible causes are:
- hidden food intolerances
- excessive toxin load
- excess overall stress burden

For possible solutions, check chapters 3, 4, and 11.

1.1 Turn off the tap

Whenever you have something that you want to improve in your health, the first thing you need to do is to stay away from things that will prevent you from achieving progress.

I call this "turning off the tap."

Imagine you have a bathtub or sink that happens to be clogged. To prevent it from overflowing, should you first...

A) start draining water as fast as possible?

OR ...

B) turn off the tap?

Most people whom I ask this question to choose correctly. Logically, "B" is the correct choice, and this applies to achieving health goals as well.

For example, if you have poor energy during the day and you choose to load up on stimulants to get an energy buzz for a few hours, that is an example of trying to "drain water" by fixing the symptoms of the problem.

Instead, if you decide to fix your digestion so you absorb nutrients that help you manage your energy levels and cell energy production, that is an example of trying to fix the "clogged bathtub," which is the true source of your problem.

Here are some examples of what to do and what not to do.

Example 1: I'm overweight. Do I…

do extra exercise after or before a meal full of highly processed starch and fats in the hope of "burning off" the excess calories?

OR…

change my meals to unprocessed, healthy meats and veggies so my body stays in fat-burning mode automatically?

Turn off the tap—Change your meals. It is almost impossible (it would take you five to six hours of physical activity per day) to "out-train" a bad diet.

Example 2: I have knee and back pain from jogging, but I love doing it. Do I …

Buy every knee guard and back brace in the physiotherapist shop so I can keep pounding the road.

OR…

Get a proper therapist to look at my injury and change my exercise routine to work around the pain and to strengthen the parts that keep being injured so they never get hurt again.

Turn off the tap—Get that injury sorted out. There are no prizes for being "gung-ho" when it comes to long-term injury, especially if you are not a professional athlete. You should get strong for the sport or activity in which you want to participate. Don't jump in too fast too soon and let that activity injure you.

Example 3: I can't seem to lose my "man boobs" and "beer belly." Do I…

try other alcoholic drinks or perhaps a "light beer"
OR...
get friends who like activities, which will help you to get closer to, not further from, your goals. Go hang out with people who like eating healthy food, climbing rock walls, lifting weights or rowing a dragon-boat for example.

Turn off the tap—Getting rid of "problem areas" can be done but not if you keep doing the same things that got you into the problem in the first place! Alcohol causes man-boobs because it requires an enzyme called alcohol dehydrogenase to detoxify in your liver.

This process depletes zinc, which is important for maintaining a good balance between male and female hormones, thus preventing a chest fat storage pattern (i.e. the less you get drunk, the less you will have to worry about a saggy chest, or buttocks for women).

I'm sure you can think of many other areas in which your life would be better if you "turned off the tap" of some habits or activities. Take a deep breath; decide to do it; find some supportive friends and get going.

1.2 Everything is a U-shaped or bell-shaped curve

In your body, almost everything is a curve. Toxins and highly processed, manmade food aside (clearly bad!), everything else is a continuum of good-to-bad-to-good, or bad-to-good-to-bad.

For example, body fat levels. An obese person almost certainly has higher risk of all kinds of diseases and health conditions. As he gets leaner, if done safely, he gets healthier. However, if he gets too lean (at something like less than 5% body fat long-term for most men, or under 10% for most women), he can develop problems.

You need fat for cell walls, energy storage, and to absorb and store fat-soluble vitamins like A, D, E, and K. You use fat for protective cushioning around organs. You also tend to have sleeping issues if body fat is too low, and there can be problems with sex hormone production, immune system weakness, and a loss of menses in women.

Another example is exercise. Certainly, a lack of exercise is a problem, but too much (quite a rare problem) can cause injury, excessive inflammation, increased stress hormone production, and sleeping irregularity.

The same thing occurs with nutrients. Vitamin C for example, too little, and you get scurvy, lowered antioxidant function and decreased immune system function. Too much, and you can get diarrhea, abdominal cramps, and increased risk of kidney stones.

I think you get the picture. In this book, the guidelines are all aimed at helping you get to that peak of the curve, while respecting your individuality. This means that the amount needed to get you to your peak will be different from the amount that others need to get them to their peak.

1.3 Long-term solutions, long-term results

Because of the "quick fix" society we live in, whether conscious or subconscious, there is a desire to get a result instantly. This is hardly ever the case, unless you are taking a pharmaceutical drug. In that case, you are getting a quick solution at the expense of passing the problem to another part of your body.

A person may want to drop 20kg (forty-four pounds) of fat right now but unless he does liposuction or is on a high dose of stimulants, appetite suppressants and fat absorption blockers, this is not going to happen. And if he does use those methods, once he stops, the weight will come back quickly as well because his body is so "shocked" by the sudden caloric restriction and weight loss that as a survival mechanism it will hold on to every ounce of food that he eats in the future as additional body fat.

However, if he uses whole foods, good sources of nutrients and lifestyle changes, his fat loss will not be as rapid but it will be sustainable and long-term. The same holds true for other physical qualities as well.

For example, when performing exercise, the hardest physical attribute to change is strength and power. It takes years of consistent, challenging and well-designed training to maximize your strength and power potential. That is why you see relatively "old" people competing in the "World's Strongest Man" competition where men aged thirty-five and up are quite a common sight.

However, people who gain strength by long-term, consistent training tend to keep it for a long time as well. Old time strongmen are often strong well into their senior years. This fact also is visible in our long-term, experienced clients. When they stop gym training for a while because of a business trip or a holiday, they come back to their previous strength levels very quickly. The longer they have been training before the break, the faster they regain their strength. Things that are slow to develop are usually also slow to lose.

Alternatively, one of the easiest physical qualities to improve is cardiovascular endurance. This can be vastly improved in a few weeks, as many runners will attest. However, it drops rapidly as well when it is not trained. Things that are fast to develop are also fast to lose.

1.4 No magical single solutions

Once again, if you want to do things for the long-term, in a healthy, natural way, it is almost impossible to get a magical, single solution to your problem. Your body is so interconnected that there is rarely a magic bullet solution to any issue.

Let's take the 20kg (forty-four pound) overweight man as an example again. Is there a single food for him to eat to get rid of all that weight? Is there a single supplement to eat? Is there a single food not to eat? Is there one magic exercise for him to do? Is there one magic late night television infomercial device that will work?

No, there is no single solution. In most cases, it is impossible to get 100% or even 50% better progress with one single form of intervention. Here is a more accurate reflection of how the body works.

The percentages can vary from person to person but the principle doesn't change.

- He stops eating refined carbohydrates—perhaps fat burning speed increases by 25%, if he performs just this one single action.
- He increases protein intake to optimal levels—increase 10%.
- He does resistance training, and interval training to boost metabolism—increase 7%.
- He takes nutrients like omega-3s, which help his cells function better as fat burning machines—increase 5%.
- He sleeps better to have more fat burning hormones released at night—increase 5%.
- He improves his digestion by removing allergenic foods—increase 3%.
- He manages stress better by removing toxins—increase 3%.
- He manages stress better by removing toxic interpersonal relationships—increase 3%.
- He becomes more relaxed by choosing to be a more grateful and positive person—increase 3%.
- He changes his water source to one that is more alkaline and filtered—increase 2%.

and so on...

In this way, he gets massive results. However, not by making one massive change—which does not exist—but rather by multiple smaller ones.

1.5 An important question to ask information providers

Often, there will be clients who come up to me and say "I read that XYZ is good for reducing the risk of cancer," or "My friend said that ABC is better for helping me lose weight," or any of a long list of possible good or bad things.

If we followed every one of these "bits" of advice, we would be jumping all over the place with little to no results to show for our efforts. Sometimes the most damaging information can be passed on by the most well-meaning people. However, when it comes to your health, your fitness and your results, it can be hard to tell the truth from the fakes especially if the intentions of the source are good.

However, here is a quick question that has helped me a lot in both business situations and in the murky waters of fitness and health information. I learned it first on an audio program by the late personal development author Napoleon Hill.

Whenever someone gives an opinion (and it is increasingly easy to hear hundreds of differing opinions on the Internet), simply ask them this one question…

Here it is…

"How do you know?"

There. It is simple; just four words. Whenever somebody with questionable intentions or knowledge is presented with this question, they will usually struggle to answer. Watch them squirm; it's entertaining…

It is a lot easier to tell if they are trying to pull a quick one on you by listening to their answer to this question, than by listening to their (perhaps rehearsed) initial statement or opinion.

If you are not convinced, ask again. "How do you know that?" until you get a satisfactory answer. If all you get in reply is: *"I read it in a magazine"* or *"I saw it on my friend's Facebook status update"* then continue checking and doing your own research

If you get "I'm a health professional. It was published in a non-commercially sponsored, peer reviewed study, and it works for a large proportion of my large client base whose progress has been tracked for months" then it's a lot more likely to be correct information and advice for you.

Try it on shady salespeople, Internet forum "gurus" who are just giving you their (usually uninformed) opinion or even a friend who may be a great friend but may not be in the best position to help you get results.

Especially in the age of Internet where opinions abound but facts are hard to find, I like the point made by author Isaac Asimov.

"Democracy means that my ignorance is just as good as your knowledge."

Therefore, even though we live in a democracy (especially online!) make sure you are getting information from those who are informed.

1.6 Mindset

I am not a big fan of "self-improvement" books and seminars in general. While I do read them, and there are some excellent ones out there, most of them target a person's enthusiastic emotions and feelings while leaving their character and actions unchanged. The correct level of love for yourself and your loved ones that is required to make changes to your habits and lifestyle is not an easy topic to address but here are some tips, along with some of the resources that I have drawn principles from that have helped my clients with their journey of change.

1.6.1 Habit formation

"Watch your thoughts, for they become words.
Watch your words, for they become actions.
Watch your actions, for they become habits.
Watch your habits, for they become character.
Watch your character, for it becomes your destiny."
—Ghandi

As Ghandi said, it starts with your thought process. You will need to sort that out and decide beforehand that health is something you want to pursue. Once you have that set, here are some tips to habit formation that will help give you long-term results.

Get a supportive community

I believe that it is impossible to overestimate the importance of the right social environment for success. After all, it has been said that in anything, *"You are the average of the five people you spend the most time with"* and this is certainly true when it comes to health.

Imagine if all your friends spent their after work hours downing pizza and beer. What do you think your chances are that you would end up like them and most likely fat and unhealthy? Pretty high!

If the opposite were true, all of your friends loved some kind of healthy activity, then even on some days when you felt a craving for cookies, or wanted to watch television instead of exercise, this community would give you a positive nudge (or shove!) forward into positive actions.

There also is the "tall poppy" syndrome in some circles where people who are trying to do something positive for themselves are taken down by jealous people around them. If people around you say things like:

"Why are you eating that kind of boring food? Come have a beer with us!

"Do you think you are better than us by trying to be so healthy? Don't be a health nut!"

"Don't you feel like you don't have a life if you eat all that healthy food?"

You really do need to get away from them. While that may sound harsh, after performing several thousand nutritional and health consultations over ten years, it is the absolute truth.

I would go one step further and actually list some people who can help you in different areas of your life, because one person is unlikely to be able to help you with everything. Having this list will greatly reduce your stress and that leads to far greater results. Who (e.g., a doctor, coach, trainer or very experienced, well-educated friend/family member) helps you with your:

- physical health?
- emotional health?
- financial health?
- spiritual health?
- accountability for change?

and so on…

Measure process goals, not results.

This idea is very well known among high achievers and top-level sportsmen and women. This is because process goals are 100% within your control, while results are not. However, the successful completion of process goals will help you achieve results.

For example, given your genetics, current health status and previous health issues, you may or may be able to reduce your body fat by 10% in three months. That is just a result. It is not entirely within your control.

However, if you plan healthy meals, regular exercise and a good amount of social support activities into your calendar, and measure how often you succeed in getting these activities completed, you are very likely to achieve your result if you score high on your "process" measurements.

In this book, you will find many "lists" of tips, or things to do. It is far better to do one or two of these things consistently for a few weeks in a row, thus building in that habit. For most habits, twenty-one days is enough to get it set as part of your life. This is a better idea than trying to do all ten things on a list then "burning out" after two or three days. The items on the lists in this book often are excellent choices for process goal setting.

If you are the kind of person who likes to visualize success, the same idea applies, visualize the successful completion of your process goals, not the results.

Prepare logistically.
Make it easier for yourself to succeed by preparation. Many distractions can stop us from achieving our desired results. So make it easier on yourself by being prepared. Keep healthy snacks available, have choices in mind for healthy restaurants and menu items so you will have something to say when your colleagues ask "Where should we go for lunch?" Keep some exercise clothes in your car so you can sneak in a workout during unexpected lull periods and so on. These simple logistic preparations help make it harder for you to give yourself excuses.

Do whatever it takes to get started.
That initial push is the hardest. That first step on the journey of a thousand miles is the hardest one. So use this principle to your advantage. Put that jar of unhealthy food far away (or better still, leave it at the store), put your computer outside your bedroom so it's more likely that you will sleep early without surfing the Internet.

Change at your own pace but move forward.
Some of our clients are highly driven, type "A" personalities who are willing and accustomed to rapid change. They can go from the pizza and beer lifestyle one day, to the veggies and free-range meats the next.

However, not everyone is like that. In fact, most people prefer gradual change. Even most research shows that changing one behavior at a time has more than double the success rate of changing two things at a time.

No problem, even if you change one or two habits per week, you will still achieve great success. The key thing, regardless of your personality, is that you change and move forward.

Actions are more important that attitude
Having a great attitude is wonderful, and probably makes you a happier person. However, in my opinion attitude is not as

important as actions. For example, there are some people who I have coached who are wonderfully pleasant people. I would like to have friends like them. However, once they hit an obstacle, or a new and challenging exercise, they tend to give up. They smile but they don't push through.

Alternatively, there are clients who whine and moan a lot when presented with a new challenge. However, they do give 110% effort once they get started. These clients get better results that the pleasant people who give up sooner.

To illustrate this further, I like the example of the airplane full of passengers who are afraid of flying, all of them are negative about flying, have a lot of fear, doubt and anxiety about the trip. Overall, they have a terrible attitude. However, does this overall, negative attitude affect the safety of the flight?

Of course not, as long as the worried passengers stay safely in their seats. It is the positive actions and training time spent by the aircraft designers, maintenance crew and well trained pilots that affect the safety of the flight.

Therefore, no matter how you feel today, this feeling is less important than taking positive actions. These actions, done consistently will "wire" your brain to make permanent changes. You need to practice taking these positive steps and you will be successful.

1.6.2 Common excuses and how to overcome them

Here are some excuses that people give and how to overcome them. These ideas are linked to **(1.6.1)** on habit formation.

I have no time.

First, we make time for things that are important to us. After all, I see people update their Facebook status at 2am and at 6am; so, clearly that is important to them. Why not spend some of that time preparing good food for the week? Why not spend it with some basic exercises at home or an early trip to the gym?

My home country of Singapore recently ranked number one in the world in "hours worked per week." True, that isn't a great thing to be number one at but that just makes preparation and planning more important and Internet surfing and television watching less important.

"Don't say you don't have enough time. You have exactly the same number of hours per day that were given to Helen Keller, Pasteur, Michelangelo, Mother Teresa, Leonardo Da Vinci, Thomas Jefferson, and Albert Einstein."
—*Life's Little Instruction Book*, compiled by **H. Jackson Brown, Jr.**

Starting a new program is difficult/intimidating, etcetera.
Get like-minded friends, social support, the right environment and perhaps even the right coach.

"Normal" people think I am weird for taking health seriously.

Remember there is a difference between normal and average. It's average to eat processed junk most of the time but that doesn't make it normal. What is normal is to take care of yourself and to eat healthy food.

You should also surround yourself with more positive and encouraging people. Having a supportive community is one of the biggest factors in long-term success.

Here are some of my common replies to statements by people who are not supportive of your health goals. Say them in a friendly but firm tone!

They say: "Oh, why do you have to eat healthy all the time? Why do you need to exercise every day? Don't be such a party popper."

You say: "Why is it that I have to explain to you the reasons that I want to eat nutritious food and have healthy habits? It's you who should have to explain to me why it's okay to sit around all day and stuff yourself with beer, cream puffs and pizza."

They say: "Why do you take nutritional supplements? Don't you know they could be dangerous, and after all, you can get all you need from food."

You say: "Why is it that there are more than a hundred thousand deaths from prescription drugs each year but almost zero from nutritional supplements? Why is it that it is okay for our plants and animals to be grown in low nutrient soil and with poor quality feed, and yet it's not okay for me to cover the missing nutrients with a supplement?"

They say: "Why do you bother to cook and bring healthy food around? I don't have time for that."

You say: "I see you updating your Facebook status at 1am on weekdays, and talking about all the television shows you watch on weekends. I think you have an hour or two per week to get some food cooked."

Finally, please remember, it is not you who needs to explain yourself to others, when what you are doing is good for your health. You being healthy means you are a better boss, employee, spouse, child or parent! It is those who eat potato chips, deep fried food and processed snacks all of the time that need to explain their behavior to you!

Eating healthy food is boring.

Most of the world eats only about fifteen different foods total most of the time. Most people eat the same old foods—just unhealthy foods. So, if you are going to be boring anyway, be healthy at least! Give this thought exercise a try, just list the foods you have eaten in the past week (e.g., rice, beef, chicken, apples, oranges, potatoes, bread)… It's not that easy to make a long list for most people!

Excuses versus changes.

One of the challenges of being a coach is that it is my job to help a person change things that he or she may not find easy to change. If it were easy to change, my coaching and mentoring role would be redundant. I would only need to teach but without a need to coach or mentor.

There are a million and one reasons that can be given for not living a healthy life. Some of them may even be "valid" excuses. However, in the bigger picture of things, whether they are valid or not, they are still excuses and it is still an individual's responsibility to choose. The choice is simple but not always easy, it's either make excuses, or make changes. I hope everyone chooses to make positive changes!

1.6.3 Success Mindset resources.

I have read literally dozens of coaching books, and if I had to choose the top three that I have found to really make a difference in the success I have had in coaching clients to achieve great results, here they are. I choose them because they are well researched, and written by authors who are interested in getting results not just an emotional high.

59 Seconds—Think A Little, Change A Lot
—by **Richard Wiseman**

This is an excellent book that is based not on feelings but on academic research of behavior change.

With Winning In Mind 3rd Edition
—by **Lanny Bassham**

I am not a fan of ineffective sports psychology. However, this book is different from that. It is written by an Olympic and world champion shooter and mental training coach. This guy knows his process goal setting and personal growth information and has gotten serious results with them both for himself and his clients. He takes a very balanced view of mind training.

Thick Face, Black Heart: The Warrior Philosophy For Conquering The Challenges Of Business And Life
—by **Chin-Ning Chu**

This is a book based on ancient Chinese wisdom quite along the lines of *The Art Of War* but very practical, it helps many people to avoid the time wasting double-mindedness associated with trying to please everyone—which is impossible anyway. It is a results-based book supported by a strong sense of logic, morals and ethics.

Chapter 2

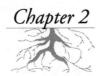

WEIGHT MANAGEMENT

M aggie was one of our clients who enjoyed competing in fitness model competitions. In an attempt to lose body fat, her previous advisors, in typical "bodybuilding fashion" had her eating a diet high in protein and very low in fat. While she did temporarily lose fat, she had longer-term issues of mood swings, yo-yo weight gain, menstrual issues and inconsistent energy levels.

It was only when she started working with a wider variety of foods including large amounts of healthy fats that she started seeing long-term improvements in her body fat levels, as well as the end of all of her health issues.

Key learning point: Work on health first, and a lean body will follow.

This chapter will cover the importance of being within a healthy weight range but far more importantly, within a healthy range of body fat. It will also cover the different methods of body fat measurement and their advantages and disadvantages.

This chapter will also cover what to do if you are overweight or underweight, and what methods will help you safely get to the shape and level of body fat you want to achieve.

2.1 What does a healthy body look like?

With all of the photo-shopped film stars and models both male and female in magazine photos these days, it can be hard to know what a healthy body shape looks like. On one hand, obesity rates keep going up across the developed world, while on the other hand, celebrities get more and more perfect looking with digital editing. For a more realistic view of the world, search for photos of actresses and models without makeup and you will have far more realistic expectations.

From experience, it's best to aim for a healthy fat percentage rather than any particular weight. It is far more important to have low body fat, and sufficient healthy lean muscle mass. In addition, low body fat is a far better indicator of health than simple weight measurements.

For a person with a regular, sedentary job but who cares a lot about their long-term health, men should aim to be between 10–12% fat year-round and women about 17–19%.

Yes, low body fat is possible if you starve yourself but the key is to achieve this goal while maintaining all of your lean mass. **(2.2)**

There are some genetic differences and some people are naturally leaner than others are but these ranges are very achievable if you have no pre-existing health issues, have very good nutrition habits and a follow proper exercise plan.

Assuming you are not a naturally lean person (most of us are not!) then these numbers will take some dedication to reach through healthy means. However, once you do reach these targets, you are very likely to have extremely good health and a great looking physique to match.

2.2 Why body fat and lean mass are your key indicators

The idea that only weight and height are important for indicating your level of health (thankfully) is regarded as old-fashioned and incomplete now. Low body fat is not only good looking but if you achieved it by healthy methods (e.g., no starvation diets or appetite suppressing pills) it also means you are far more likely to have good insulin sensitivity (9.9) and lower risk of lifestyle diseases like diabetes, cardiovascular conditions and some forms of cancer. Most notably, cancer of the:

- esophagus,
- pancreas,
- colon and rectum,
- breast (after menopause),
- endometrium (lining of the uterus),
- kidney,
- thyroid, or
- gallbladder.

Maintaining or increasing lean mass (muscles) while you burn off fat is critical. Lean mass boosts metabolism, improves your immune system so you fall sick less often and is an important factor in high quality of life especially as people age. All of those studies that show that a person loses lean mass as they age are accurate only for sedentary people but they don't apply to people who do a consistent strength training program (12.3, 12.4).

Alternatively, if a person focuses on weight alone, and achieves lower weight with excessive, long cardiovascular exercise, and a long-term low calorie diet, he or she is likely to lose a lot of lean mass and will not reap the benefits listed above. In addition, there is an almost 100% certainty of regaining that weight "with interest" because long-term food restriction sets up muscle loss, lowered metabolism and a hormone driven urge to binge eat and store fat.

2.3 Methods of body fat measurement—which is best?

To track the progress of your training and nutrition program, you need a way to track your body fat accurately.

If it goes down, you are on the right track, and if it does not, or goes up, you need to make some modifications. However, not all fat measurement methods are created equal. Here are some common and not so common ones. From the pros and cons, you will be able to choose a method that suits you best.

What is BMI? Why is it not great but yet very popular?

It can be very difficult to assess the health of a large group of people. It might be impossible or excessively time consuming to get all of the right data all the time.

One such case is when studying obesity and health related issues. The standard measurement is the Body Mass Index or BMI. It's an ancient formula from the 1800s, and it is mass in kilos, divided by height in meters squared. So if you were 80kg and 170cm tall, it would be $80/(1.7*1.7) = 27.68$

This can be done by anybody with a primary school math education and because of its simplicity, it is often used in population studies of health. However, is it the best for you? I would say, probably not.

Here are three reasons why you should consider using body-fat percentage as a better gauge of health (assuming you got to a healthy percentage by a healthy lifestyle, not liposuction, or anabolic steroids).

- You can have a "healthy" BMI while still being fat. I call this "skinny-fat" and it is a problem for many men and women.
- It leads to an obsession with weight, rather than health, especially among women.
- It leads to men being considered "overweight" even if they are actually lean, strong, fit and muscular, as most lean, fit people will fall into the overweight or even obese zones of the BMI chart.

It underestimates the number of people who are "over-fat." In a recent study, BMI estimated the number of obese people at 23% but with a far more accurate DEXA scan, the amount of people who were over-fat was 64%.

BMI—Body mass index

- Pros: Very simple to do and great for big studies with hundreds of people because it can be calculated fast.
- Cons: Incomplete picture. Not so useful to each individual because it assumes a fat and weak person as the norm.

Even a moderately sized person who weighs 73kg at 170cm height would be overweight. Any male who exercises regularly can achieve that size. Some people are genetically thicker and bigger. BMI does not account for this either.

Here is just one of many examples of how BMI may not lead to accurate conclusions. Both of these clients of mine were measured at 78kg and about 178cm tall. They have exactly the same BMI but one is at 22% fat and one is at 8%. Which physique is healthier? The answer is quite obvious. The second picture is the typical "skinny-fat" look. While the first picture is extremely lean and muscular, yet natural, a look that most people both male and female would prefer.

Circumference measurements

What is it? Measuring the circumference around different parts of the body. There are variations of this method measuring waistline at smallest point, waist at belly button, arms, thighs, wrists etcetera.

- Pros: Quite easy to do as long as you get the points right, and if you use a good measuring tape called a Gullick tape that uses a spring to consistently get the same tension in the tape.
- Cons: Does not take bone structure into account, and can vary from time to time (e.g., if you just had a meal, or a bottle

of water, your waist would go up even though your fat level did not).

Fat measurement scales and handheld devices

What is it? It is usually an electrical impedance device that uses electric current to see how easily it passes through your body. In theory, it should pass through muscle better because muscle has more water content than fat, and water conducts electricity.

- Pros: Simple to use—hold the handles, or step on the footpads, and press start.
- Cons: Wild fluctuations in measurements. This is because these use electrical methods, which rely on your body's current hydration status in specific areas of the body. This can change if you drink, eat, sit, stand, are in different parts of a menstrual cycle, sweat, etcetera. Accuracy tends to be plus or minus 7%. That is too much variance to know if you are close to an ideal amount, or not. For example, if a person was 14%, he may measure at 7% (professional athlete) or 21% (sedentary office worker).

Caliper measurements

What is it? Use of a set of calipers to take measurements of skinfolds at different parts of the body, then using a research-based formula to get an approximate body fat reading. There can be different formulas using as few as one skinfold site to as many as twelve.

- Pros: Very accurate if done right by a good practitioner with good equipment. For lean people, they can be almost as accurate as a DEXA scan.
- Cons: Needs a lot of constant practice to do properly. It is like playing a musical instrument. Literally thousands of measures before it becomes "second nature" and consistently correct.

Hydrostatic weighing

What is it? You sit in a water-filled device and it measures the amount of water you displace. When matched to your weight, you can see if you displace a lot or a little water for your weight. If you displace a lot, that means you are fatter because fat is less dense than muscle.

- Pros: Accurate and good for general population
- Cons: May not be as accurate for other populations (e.g. athletes and elderly). This is because they have different bone and muscle densities that are not taken into account by the standard formulas

DEXA scan

What is it? It stands for "dual-energy X-ray absorptiometry" this means that two x-rays are used, a high-energy one, and a low-energy one. The different X-rays are absorbed differently by different body tissues and the readings can show how much of each tissue you have.

- Pros: Good accuracy if the same machine is used, can give readings of not only total amount but also where the fat is distributed (e.g., fat around organs is more damaging to health).
- Cons: It is an x-ray and repeated radiation exposure is not a good idea, thus should not be done often. There can also be differences between machines and brands.

Photographs

- Pros: Anybody can do it with cameras being so commonplace
- Cons: It takes effort to get consistency. The photo must be taken at the same time, same day of the week, same camera, same tripod, same location, same lighting conditions, etcetera. It is these variables that marketing companies use to sell "magical" before and after pictures of fitness products.

2.3.1 Suggested method

The most practical method if you were alone would probably be circumference measurements. However, because that is not as accurate, it may be worth it to get professionally measured occasionally by either:

- a skilled practitioner with calipers, or
- a DEXA scan/hydrostatic weighing.

There are some medical clinics that have DEXA scans or hydrostatic pods for about $200 per measurement.

If you choose the calipers route, here are some ways to tell if the person knows what he or she is doing, which will help you get an accurate result.

- Use good calipers. The cheap white plastic ones are not accurate enough for professional use. A good caliper can cost more than $400 USD. However, good calipers such as Harpenden are accurate to 0.2mm and can even help a skilled practitioner see if you are retaining water.
- They measure fat often as part of their job, every day if possible.
- They use at least a seven-site formula. A twelve-site bio-signature formula is even better and more useful for detecting problem areas.
- They pinch your fat HARD and get ALL of it using a wide grip (not two fingers). The common mistake I see many practitioners make is they are afraid to cause discomfort to the client/patient. Sorry, if you are overly fat, it may be uncomfortable for a few seconds when your fat is being pinched. However, you want an accurate result, right?
- They try to measure at the same time of the day.
- They don't measure you after long flights.
- They can tell you what to do to improve your results once you get them.

Even if you choose a less than perfect measure, as long as you try to be as consistent with all the variables, it can still give you a useful and meaningful result. There is a saying, "You can't manage what you can't measure" and measuring body fat is certainly going to help you manage it with a lifestyle, nutrition and exercise program.

2.4 How to know if a weight loss method is a scam?

Just like investing money, weight loss is a very emotional and personal topic so there is a lot of room for over-hyped products, or unethical businesses to take advantage of people. Here are some ways to tell if a diet or workout program is a weight loss scam.

It recommends extremely low calories.

If you follow one of these starvation plans, your body's metabolism will eventually shut down to adjust to the low food intake. This is the way to look sickly and thin, rather than fit, healthy and radiant.

It recommends extremely low fat.

If a diet plan tells you to avoid fat like the plague, it is bad for you. Fat is critical for many important processes in your body **(9.1)**. If you don't eat fat, you can quite literally die! The logic is slightly counter-intuitive but allow me to use some real life experiences to which you can relate.

Can you recall a day when you were too busy, or stressed or simply didn't have a chance to drink enough water? I'm sure you probably can, and on that day, did you urinate more or less? Less for sure! Why? Because when you lack something, your body tries as much as possible to hold on to what you have, in this case, water.

The same principle applies to burning fat as well. You need to eat fat to burn fat. In the nutrition section we will talk about what kinds, and how much but for now, just know that making everything "low fat" is a bad idea.

It focuses only on weight loss and not on fat loss.
If the marketing and testimonials only say how much weight a person loses, think twice about joining that program. Either they are not tracking fat loss, or they don't think it's important. Both are bad signs.

It does not focus on maintaining or increasing lean mass.
As described above **(2.2)**, having good levels of lean mass is extremely important for long-term health. If a program does not track this, and does not place an emphasis on strength, then it is less likely to give you a long-term, high quality result.

**It promises incredible weight loss
results in an unrealistically short time.**
Just like there are "get rich quick" scams, there are also "get skinny quick" scams. These appeal to people because of the emotional attachment to both money and losing weight. We want it now!

The truth is, the more overweight you are, the faster you can drop weight safely. However, once you get within five to ten kilograms of your target weight, slowly dropping one-half to one kilogram of fat per week is the way to go.

In general, you can go for fast weight loss for a short time, or slower loss for a longer time. You can over-train, and starve yourself to drop weight fast but in such a situation your body perceives this sudden lack of food, and excess activity as an added stress, and this actually stimulates long-term metabolism damage and extra fat storage. Long slow results are more permanent **(1.3)**.

It involves a multi-level-marketing (MLM) business model.
Some MLMs actually have decent products; however, they are not a good value buy for you, the consumer. It is a far better value to get medical grade products from reputable manufacturers **(9.8)**.

Why? Simply look at the business model; it is based on many layers of sales people. There is always a fee that has to be paid to distributors but now you have to pay many levels of commissions and fees. Mathematically, product costs ends up at about 8% of the price you pay.

With high quality, non-MLM supplements, product costs are about 20-25%. That is a lot more money in the product, rather than in salesperson's commissions, which means more quality for you, the consumer.

2.5 I need to make a change in my body; what should I do?

Recognize that you will need to change your habits and behavior.

You are totally responsible for where you are now, and your actions have led you to the state you are in currently. If you want to get a different result than what you are getting now, you will need to change your habits.

Make it "necessary" to make the change, rather than "nice."

It's easy to do something healthy for a few days but to make it a lifestyle you have to believe that health is a necessity not just another nice thing to have.

Do it out of love, not discipline.

Love is the strongest emotion in the world, and things done out of love (rather than discipline or guilt) give the most benefits (e.g., you eat healthy food because you love your health more than you love extra chocolate cake).

Understand that having the right nutrition will be very important **(Chapter 9.6.2)**. You can never out-exercise bad food choices **(9.10.6)**.

Understand that exercise is the key to maintaining lean mass as you burn fat.

You can eat well, and you will already get great benefits but proper exercise makes you look and feel awesome at the end of the process

Take action now, on what you can,
and continue making adjustments later.

You may or may not make huge changes in your life all at once. Some people do well with wholesale "cold-turkey" changes, while some people do better with gradual changes. However, the key is to make changes and keep making them until you have all the good lifestyle habits in place.

2.6 Weight management principles

Actually, it's not that complicated! From a scientific perspective, the basics of burning fat will never change. It is far more likely to be an implementation problem than a lack of information. The relevant sections in this book will help you take action on the relevant information.

- Eat a diet of unprocessed foods, low in refined carbohydrates, and high in healthy fats, veggies and proteins. Don't worry too much about the amount of food at first. Get the food choices correct. Our nutrition section in **(Chapter 9)** will help you do this.
- Use an exercise program based on strength training and interval training. **(Chapter 12)** should cover all the basics and give you something you can do today.

2.7 Some weight loss obstacles

However, there are people who do the basics and still have trouble getting to a healthy weight and body fat percentage. In cases like this there needs to be a bit of detective work done to find out exactly what is the obstacle getting in the way of good results.

You usually don't hear these reasons because they go beyond the usual "eat less and exercise more" thinking in most places. However, if you have been frustrated with your lack of results, one of these problems may be the one you need to fix to keep progressing.

Problem 1: Overtraining

While most people lack physical activity, it is possible to have "too much" of a good thing. Excessive training that you are unable to recover from places stress not only on your muscles and joints but also on your adrenal glands, which control much of your body's response to stress.

A lot of exercise combined with the stresses of work, study, and even environmental pollution can overwhelm the body's defenses and lead to a state of fat storage. This is because excess, long-term exposure to stress encourages your body to go into "survival mode" (i.e., store fat just in case we get into a starvation situation).

I know this is not likely in food abundant developed countries but that is the way our bodies deal with stress and we can't change it. So what can we do?

- Get better, deeper sleep through better nutrition (i.e., eat only unprocessed food—no grains, diary or soy, which are common allergens and add to stress)
- Use supplements like magnesium, which aids muscle relaxation and stress management in your body
- Use shorter exercise sessions never going past thirty or forty minutes.

Problem 2: Too many toxins

It is an impossible task to stay totally "toxin free" as the world gets more and more polluted. The nonprofit research group the "Environmental Working Group" did tests on the blood of newborn babies who have not even breathed polluted air. Even children born in clean parts of the world like Alaska or the remote Pacific Islands, had multiple toxins and chemicals. This is even more likely in a city or agricultural environment.

The problem is that your body will slow its metabolism when it is under a toxic load to protect itself from circulating the toxin. This makes fat burning very difficult! One simple thing you can do is to check your hair and skin care products for things like parabens and phthalates, which can disrupt your hormonal system.

Another thing you can do is to take a few grams per day (three to four grams) of the amino acid glycine, which aids your body in detoxifying petrochemicals. This should be cheaply available in most nutrition shops. If you want a great book on toxicity, the best one I have found is *Achieving Victory Over A Toxic World* by Mark Schauss.

Problem 3: Not tracking your habits

Information is not usually a problem; after all, everyone knows that grilled fish with vegetables is a better meal than potato chips. However, we may not actually know how "off track" we are when it comes to having healthy habits.

For food, aim for nine out of ten healthy meals. Therefore, if you eat a meal of non-processed, nutritious food, it's a pass. If you skipped a meal or ate refined food (e.g. bread, white rice, cookies, etcetera) that is a fail. If you get nine out of ten passes, you are well on the way to good results. Any less than that, and you have room for improvement.

For exercise, you also need to track your progress. You may not need to go for more training but if last week you took twenty minutes to run four kilometers, this week you need to be aiming for nineteen and a half minutes. If you lifted 50kg ten times last week, this week you should be aiming for 51kg or eleven repetitions. If you don't try to progress, you won't, and you will get no further results. **(Chapter 12)** will get you on track.

For sleep, you should have no more than one night per week with disturbed sleep. Not being able to fall asleep, waking up in the middle of the night and waking up feeling unrefreshed means you need to work on your sleep quality. Check out **(Chapter 3)** for sleep tips.

Chapter 3

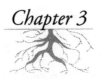

SLEEP

My personal story: Every male citizen in our country is required to perform two years of national service. During my time in the army, I was selected to attend officer training school. This was a tough nine months of continual training and sleep deprivation. We often went with five or less hours of sleep per night. My "record" was three days without sleep, by that time I was hallucinating and sleeping on my feet. In fact, I was punished with extra guard duty because I was so sleepy that an instructor stole a part of my machine gun from right under my nose. I was sleeping when I thought I was awake!

After this stressful time, I have had sleep problems and energy level issues ever since. It took me a wide variety of treatments from high levels of nutrients, clean sleep conditions, and other alternative therapies to utilize my sleep hormones better before I could sleep normally again.

Key Learning Point: Manage your stress or else sleep will suffer and health will too.

This chapter will cover the importance of sleep and what you can do with your lifestyle, environment, nutrition and other factors if you have trouble sleeping, or feel you are not having optimal energy.

Sleep is critical to health, happiness and productivity. I don't think any health professional would disagree with that! In fact, research on the parts of the brain that sleep deprivation affects shows that if you lack sleep, you are less likely to be happy because a lack of sleep affects happy thoughts and memories the most. In the study, sleep deprived participants remembered negative words and pictures far better than they did positive ones.

Unfortunately, however, "go and sleep more" doesn't work all the time for many people. From our client records, I would say that approximately 75% of the clients I have consulted with start out with less than optimal sleep patterns.

What is optimal? seven to nine hours straight with no interruptions, no waking up to pee, no trouble falling asleep (out within a couple of minutes of lying down) and waking up with high morning energy ready and excited to face the day. These are signs of good and restful sleep. If you are not getting great sleep, you increase the risk of developing all kinds of problems, including increased speed of aging, heart disease, diabetes, weight gain, inflammation and cancer. Many important immune system, detoxification and hormonal functions happen when we sleep. If you are not detoxifying, not producing the right amounts of the right hormones and weakening your immune function, things do not look good for long-term health. So what can you do about it?

The good news is that many of the things you can do to improve your sleep are cheap and effective. Here are some of the tips I give my clients to improve sleep without resorting to sleeping pills and other relaxant drugs with their negative effects and the cycle of needing "uppers" and stimulants in the morning, and "downers" and sleep inducing medication at night.

3.1 General Sleep Tips

Just as we wash our hands before we eat or brush our teeth before bed for hygiene purposes, I call the following steps that you can take before climbing into bed "sleep hygiene." They help make your sleep clean and healthy.

- **Get a pair of earplugs and eye mask.** We are designed to sleep in a quiet and dark environment. However, in most developed countries, this is extremely unlikely unless you live in a massive house with a large garden around it, off the main road, with quiet neighbors and dark curtains in your room. Since the chances of that are slim to none, get these simple and cheap sleeping aids.

- **Get your sleep area in order.** Just as you clean your teeth and your body, you need to clean up your sleep for good health. Turn off the Wi-Fi router in your room, no laptops, no cell phones, no television, no lights. We all have a different tolerance for electromagnetic and radiation stress but it certainly affects us negatively and nobody benefits from more of it.

- "Oh but my cell phone is my alarm,…" Well, get a five dollar battery-operated alarm clock instead. Be especially careful if you live in an older building, which may have faulty wiring, which leads to "dirty electricity." A Graham Stetzer filter along with a current meter to check which power points need filters, is a good idea for you. Check them out at electrahealth.com

- **Support your sleep nutritionally.** The first and most important supplement is magnesium. Everyone is deficient in this mineral. It used to be in our foods but with most of our foods produced with artificial fertilizers, it is no longer found there in sufficient amounts. Take up to two grams for men and 1.2 grams for women. Make sure the magnesium is a good quality brand to avoid loose stools **(9.8.1)**.

- **Check your overall stress levels.** In my experience, the main cause of this that people miss is found in their food in the form of subclinical food intolerances **(3.3)**. Clean up your digestion **(4.1)** and stop eating foods that your body can't tolerate. This should lower your overall stress load, and allow for better sleep.
- **Add melatonin.** Many people use this as the number one option. However, I don't recommend it. The reason is that, from my experiences using it with clients, it loses effectiveness over time, usually within one week. So use it only when you really can't sleep because of serious stresses in life, if you are working a shift job (take it just before sleep no matter what time your shift ends) or when you are recovering from jet lag.

3.2 What if I can't fall asleep?

If all of the above do not help your sleep, you may need to do some laboratory testing **(10.1)** to find out what nutrients are out of balance in your body and which biochemical reactions are not functioning well. The main test would be an organic acid test, along with a food intolerance test. A urine-based neurotransmitter test also is a good choice to see what is going on with your brain chemistry.

Another problem that you are trying to fix is excessive stress hormones in the evening. This can be a sign of adrenal fatigue **(2.5)**. In addition, there are herbs that are known to reduce stress levels and enable sleep. I only recommend medical grade supplements for my clients **(9.8)**. Most herb-based products work through management of your adrenal glands and are best used in rotation. Get several products and use each of them for a week at the recommended dosage, tracking which one works best for you. Here is a combination of herb-based products, which I have used with good results for clients.

Ashwaganda from Wise Woman Herbals
MyoCalm P.M. from Metagenics

Adreset from Metagenics
Wind Down from Poliquin

In addition, in my experience, it is important to look at what kind of training program you are on now, and what time of the day you choose to do exercise. Hard, heavy training late in the evening can disrupt sleep patterns for some clients. A combination of glycine, magnesium and phosphatidyl serine has often helped clients who face this problem.

3.3 Here are some stress busting tips

Stress is an "overall" load. In fact, your body only has a few responses to stress. These responses are the same, no matter the cause of the stress. So, in many respects, a stressful work environment will be quite similar to eating food that your body is intolerant to or your body living in a polluted environment. The response to all of these will involve the release of stress hormones, which cause havoc with the brain, immune system, fat burning and overall health.

One of the best overall books for learning about how your body handles stress is called *Why Zebras Don't Have Ulcers* by Robert Sapolsky. He is a very interesting writer, especially for a highly decorated biology professor, and he really gets some excellent points across about stress.

Because excess stress levels can be a major cause of sleep problems, here are some tips that I have found to be effective in helping clients get better quality, deeper and more restful sleep. Boosting their overall health and allowing them to reach their health goals sooner.

Tip 1: **Remove the stressor.**
Get away from whatever is causing you stress.
Tip 2: **Improve Sleep Quality (3.1, 3.2), and sleep by 10pm.**
Tip 3: **Remove Toxins.**
Toxins are an additional burden to your body. Any time you are toxic, your body responds by slowing your

metabolism (increasing fat storage). This is another survival mechanism because a slow metabolism means the toxins circulate more slowly in your body and cause less overall damage.

The most common source of toxins for women tends to come from personal care products like shampoos and makeup. Make sure your products do not carry stuff like lead, parabens, sodium lauryl sulphate and propylene glycol. Try to get natural herbal products that help you look and smell great without disrupting your fat burning. **(Chapter 10)** has more information on detoxification.

Tip 4:   **Relax your breathing.**

Correct breathing turns on the correct nervous system responses you want in your body to stay relaxed and in the right position. Because of continual stress at work and in life, most of us tend to stay in a chronically tense state. This is reflected in breathing through our mouth, and into our chest. When a person is stressed or scarred or startled (imagine being frightened by a wild animal), we "gasp" and breath through our mouth, and into our chest, activating the fight or flight response.

Instead, in most situations (except high intensity exercise or fear), we should breathe in through our nose and into our tummy. You may be surprised how "hard" this is at first if you have been breathing through your chest for much of your life. But with practice, your breathing habits can change.

The best way to learn this is by lying face up on a bench or bed. From this position, place a light object like a small book on your tummy. When you breathe, use your nose, and breathe into your tummy so the book rises up and breathe out through your mouth so the book goes down. If you do this wrong, you will use your chest and the book will hardly move at all.

Practice this lying down as it is the easiest way to learn. Once you can make the book go up and down, then start to integrate the chest into the breathing. Breathe in (nose) to tummy, then once the tummy is full, continue breathing in to fill the chest. Exhale gently through your mouth.

Tip 5: Watch what type and the amount of your exercise.

Exercise is excellent for stress management but there can be a case of too much of a good thing.

In general, if you perform heavy strength training with big weights in the evening, your nervous system may not be able to calm down in time to sleep well. If your schedule allows, shift heavy training to mornings, and check the nutrient recommendations in (3.2).

There is another possibility where people who love exercise but do too much for their recovery ability. This can overload their stress management systems. Massive amounts of exercise with moderate loads can make you over-trained by the total volume of exercise. In this case, take a week off or a de-load week at half the amount of exercise you normally do, and see if that improves your sleep. Aerobic training done in excess also is a cause of this kind of stress.

I have seen clients with both cases mentioned above, so change your exercise habits and you should also see some benefits in how easily you fall asleep.

Tip 6: Keep a grateful log.

Every day, write a journal, three things you are thankful for, something you learned, and something with which you helped someone. This helps a lot with stress management.

Tip 7: Stay away from caffeine.

This can add additional burden to your stress glands. Coffee is not bad for you but if you are already under a lot of stress, it can add more.

Tip 8: Avoid multi-tasking.
> The constant switching of your brain from one subject to another does induce a higher stress load on your hormonal system.

Tip 9: Avoid refined foods.
> Poor quality, un-natural foods increase the body's stress load.

Tip 10: Add salt to the diet.
> Do this unless you already have hypertension (high blood pressure).

3.4 What if I wake up during the night?

The stress busting tips from **(3.3)** should help you greatly in improving sleep quality. However, some people may face specific problems of waking up consistently at the same time of the night.

The solution to solving these problems usually is determined by what time your wake-up occurs. As coach Charles Poliquin teaches in his excellent bio-signature courses.

If you wake up shortly after going to sleep, the most common cause is reactive hypoglycemia, which means you don't eat enough of the right foods at the right times during the day. Follow the guidelines in the nutrition section **(9.1)** and you should have this sorted out.

If you wake up at 1-3am, it's often a liver related issue. Cut down on your liver stress with nutrients that support your liver. As well as reducing the stress on your liver from alcohol and other toxins. In my experience, people who have a high alcohol intake face this problem with greater frequency. The nutrients that support liver processes are covered in **(10.2)**.

If you wake up at 3-5am, the most common cause of this is a low antioxidant level for your current needs **(5.5.3)**. Everyone has different needs depending on your genetics, lifestyle and stresses. An increase in antioxidants via foods or supplementation will help you out here.

Also check out your waking environment, is there a lot of loud noise or activity in your neighborhood? Is there a great deal of sunlight suddenly entering your room **(3.1)**?

3.5 What if I have low morning energy?

Unfortunately, I have found from our lifestyle consultations that low morning energy is the norm for most people but that doesn't mean it's normal! Assuming you are able to sleep well and for at least seven to eight hours each night, you will need to consider what is known as adrenal fatigue as a possible cause of your low energy.

The best book I have found on this is called *Adrenal Fatigue: The 21st Century Stress Syndrome* by Dr. James Wilson. Go to the website www.adrenalfatigue.org and take the online questionnaire. It should give an indicator of how fatigued your adrenals are.

A good laboratory test is a saliva adrenal stress index test, which uses saliva taken every four hours to see the changes you have in stress hormones thought the day. Adrenal fatigue usually is categorized into seven stages. With one being the least serious and seven being the most serious.

Which stage of adrenal fatigue are you in?

Stage 1: Cortisol (i.e. stress hormones) and sex hormones are high.
Symptoms: not many.

Stage 2: Cortisol goes even higher, sex hormones drop.
Symptoms: disruption in sleep patterns, digestive issues, random aches and pains.

Stage 3: Sex hormones continue to drop as raw material is being used for cortisol production.
Symptoms: Exhaustion, anxiety.

Stage 4: Can't wake up in the morning because cortisol is being used later in the day.

Symptoms: Difficulty waking up and staying up, sleep very disrupted as blood sugar drops, difficulty falling asleep (become a "night person").

Stage 5: Very tired in the afternoon, almost bedridden.

Stage 6: Very tired during the whole day.

Stage 7: Tired all day and can't get motivated to do anything.

If this is you, then a good functional medicine doctor will be able to help you get over these problems. From my experience, Stage 1 to 3 or 4 can often be dealt with by yourself by simply taking stress management steps **(3.3)**, and taking health seriously as described in this book. However, treatment for anything from Stage 4 onward should be under some form of supervision from a health care professional.

The general period for a good functional doctor to help you from Stage 7 back to Stage 1 is about twelve months. This is a long time, so the best choice is to manage your stress levels continually so you don't get to Stage 7. In fact, anything past Stage 4 is very serious; most people notice issues starting at Stage 3.

The reason I suggest a professional for a more complex situation is because there is a lot going on which can lead to adrenal fatigue symptoms, and each person can have similar symptoms, but with different root causes of their problems.

The low adrenal function can be caused by multiple factors which can start "higher up" in the hormone chain, in an area of your brain called the hypothalamus, and in another place called the pituitary gland. Circulating levels of other hormones, brain chemicals, and immune system function can be part of the whole situation that you may need to deal with.

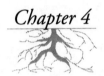

Chapter 4

DIGESTION

L indsey was one of the clients at our gym, and she was one of the most promising young golfers in our country. However, she was underweight and her lack of strength was limiting her progress at golf. During our initial interview, we found out that her digestive system was not in good shape. She had bloating after meals, as well as being constipated, and passed stool only once every seven to ten days. After a gut-rebuilding program using the steps shown below, she was able to pass stools daily and eat more without bloating. Within fifteen weeks, she gained 5kg of lean mass and had vastly improved strength. None of this would have been possible if we had not first addressed her digestive tract issues.

Key point: It's not just what you eat; it's what you are able to absorb that makes all the difference.

This chapter will cover the importance of digestive health and how it affects almost all other areas of health from weight loss, to sleeping disorders. A basic plan for digestive health will be outlined, as well as more advanced methods of testing for and fixing digestive healthy issues.

4.1 Digestion basics: What's actually happening in there? What can go wrong?

Our digestive tract or "gut" is amazing. It takes food of all types, nutrient content, vitamin and mineral content, shapes and sizes, separates it out, breaks it all down and makes it ready to use as energy, while at the same time making sure that any toxins or bacteria don't harm you.

If your gut is messed up, you are likely to have symptoms like diarrhea, constipation, acid reflux, bloated feelings after food that takes a long time to go away and even memory and mood problems. Why such a wide range of problems? Because your gut provides a wide range of services!

Aside from digestion, which you probably already know about, it also performs nervous system functions of producing two thirds of your brain chemicals so it's critical for brain health and brain function too **(6.1)**.

Your digestive tract also performs advanced immune system function, estimated at 70% of your body's total immune function. It also has a huge surface area exposed to the environment for good absorption of nutrients (approximately $400m^2$, an area slightly less than two entire tennis courts) but this exposure means it's vulnerable to toxins and bacteria, so the immune system in the gut needs to be functioning at a high level as well.

Because it performs such a wide variety of important functions, the digestive tract is an excellent starting point to work on almost all health conditions. Most functional doctors would agree that when in doubt about what to do with a chronic health problem, fix the gut first.

4.2 Simple steps to digestive health

Before you start, you need to know if your digestion is indeed compromised. The simplest and quickest tests are the three shown below. If you don't do well on them, chances are, a serious look at your digestive tract is in order.

Test 1: The zinc taste test

This test is well-documented (British Medical Association's British National Formulary 1988) as a safe, cheap and accurate indication of zinc status in your body. To do this test you will need a teaspoon of zinc sulphate solution.

It's pretty cheap and I use the Metagenics, Designs For Health, or Poliquin brand testing liquid. You put the teaspoon of the clear liquid into your mouth and swish it around in your mouth for approximately ten seconds. Go ahead and swallow, wait thirty seconds, then rate the aftereffects on a scale of 1 to 4.

1. Optimal zinc level—Immediate, unpleasant, obvious taste that makes you want to spit out the liquid.
2. Adequate zinc level—Definite but not strongly unpleasant taste immediately, which intensifies with time but not so bad that it makes you want to spit.
3. Moderate zinc deficiency—No taste initially but mild taste after ten to fifteen seconds.
4. Very zinc deficient—tastes like water (tasteless).

If you do poorly on this test, a zinc supplement would be of great benefit to you, and you will probably need a vitamin B6 and magnesium supplement as well as these three nutrients work together. Vitamin B6 is needed to transfer zinc and magnesium to cells.

Test 2: *The stomach acid test*

Note: The best test for stomach acid is probably the Heidelberg stomach acid test. But this requires a trip to the hospital and costs between 300-500 USD. So the one I am recommending is the one you can do at home for a tiny fraction of the cost.

Safety: Don't do this test if you currently have peptic ulcers, or are currently on NASID anti-inflammatory medication. If you are in doubt please check with your doctor to see if your medication increases the risk of gastritis. For everyone else, it's a safe test because it's just a mild addition to the digestive acid that your stomach already produces.

Stomach hydrochloric acid (HCL) is a very critical part of health because adequate levels of HCL are needed to:

- digest protein properly (undigested protein just rots!),
- kills bacteria,
- activates enzymes, hormones and brain chemicals (neurotransmitters), and
- aids in absorption of essential minerals and antioxidants.

It just doesn't make sense to work on healthy nutrition and supplements if you can't absorb them well because of low HCL levels. That would be a complete waste of time and money.

To do this test you will need to test with a portion of meat. I would suggest at least a palm-sized portion. This is because solid protein is the most challenging thing to digest and protein digestion benefits most from good levels of HCL.

- On the next meal that you have, eat half of the meat portion and then take one, two-hundred milligram capsule of HCL.

- Continue with the rest of your meal, and wait five to fifteen minutes
- If your stomach acid levels are adequate, you will feel a warm, "burning" sensation in your chest. Don't worry it's not dangerous, and if it is very uncomfortable, take a glass of water to get rid of the feeling.
- If your stomach acid is insufficient, you will feel nothing.
- If you feel nothing, on the next meal you have meat, have two capsules of HCL instead of one. Again, wait for the burning, warm feeling.
- If you get it, you should take one capsule (the highest dose at which you do NOT get the warm feeling) at each meal to aid your digestion
- If you do not get the warm feeling, continue adding to the dosage each meal until you reach seven capsules (or fourteen-hundred milligrams), or get the warm feeling. Back off by one capsule to get the right dose for your current needs (e.g., if you get the feeling at four capsules, your current dose needed is three capsules).
- Continue with HCL supplementation until your digestion improves. As you improve, you will start to get the warm feeling with your current dose, and you can reduce the dose by one capsule.

Test 3: The poop test

You will need three cups of cooked corn (because it's easy to see in your poop). Consume it at your last meal of the day. Then you will need to take note of the first and the last time that you can see corn in your poop. The normal times should be between eighteen and twenty-two hours after the meal.

If it's too fast and diarrhea-like, the probiotic SB (saccharomyces boulardii) is a good way to fix that.

Take one capsule three times per day.

And if it's too slow/constipated, make sure hydration is adequate (at least four liters of water per day for an 80kg man), take 500 to 1000mg of vitamin C three times per day with meals, along with 500 to 1500mg of magnesium glycinate before bed has shown good results with clients and should get things smoothly again.

What if I fail these tests?

Take a combination of these three tests, and if you don't do well on them, go through the four "R"s below and get your gut sorted out before trying to work on the rest of your health issues. They are the four "R"s about which gut experts always talk. Remove, Replace, Re-inoculate, Repair. Just follow them and your chances of a healthier gut will be a lot higher!

Step 1: Remove allergenic foods.

Your gut has a very good protective wall that only allows good stuff into your blood and sends bad stuff out of your backside. Allergenic foods damage this wall and allow undigested food and toxic material into circulation. So getting rid of foods that irritate the protective wall is critical.

If you are sensitive, you can sometimes tell which foods you are sensitive to by mild physical reactions. In this case we are talking about a subclinical allergy. So, you are not going to go into shock and stop breathing; however, you may get mild symptoms such as watery eyes, itchy ears or skin, runny nose, sneezing, waking up in the middle of the night, and low energy for no particular reason.

These symptoms usually come within a few hours but may take as long as two days. However, if you are aware of what to look for, and can recall what you have eaten, you can often pick out some possible suspects.

In my experience with hundreds of clients per year, as well as with a lot of food allergy lab tests **(10.1)** for clients, these are the common foods that can cause problems for people's guts. In reality, it could be anything, and I have had clients who have been intolerant of "healthy" foods such as broccoli, celery and tomatoes. However, this is much more rare. Work on the common "problem foods" first.

Common food allergens:

- milk,
- wheat,
- gluten,
- eggs (white or yolk),
- peanuts,
- soy products, and
- other nuts (not often all kinds but one or two e.g. cashews or almonds for a particular person).

Be aware any time you eat the above foods and if you suspect something, don't eat it for six weeks or so. After that, add it back into the system and check for the symptoms. They are often easier to detect because you tend to have a more "violent" reaction after being off the food for a while. If you are okay with the food, it's probably okay for you to eat it again.

As a rule as well, try to rotate your foods. Human beings generally only eat about fifteen to twenty different foods most of the time, and the more often you eat something, the more likely you are to get sensitivity to it **(9.1)**. If you find a lot of sensitive foods, your gut is likely compromised and its best to get your food allergens checked with laboratory testing **(10.1)**.

Step 2: Replace missing digestive elements.
In this case, the most likely things to be missing from your digestive tract are hydrochloric acid, and digestive enzymes. A HCL supplement, as well as a broad-based digestive enzyme formula should help you here.

Step 3: Re-inoculate yourself with good bacteria.

There is a constant war between good and bad bacteria in your digestive tract. If the bad bacteria are winning it's called "disbiosis" and you get symptoms like:

- more allergies of all kinds,
- poor nutrition absorption and thus nutrient deficiencies,
- constipation,
- chronic diarrhea,
- respiratory infection,
- cognitive (brain) problems,
- weight gain, skin conditions because of poor detoxification,
- your blood does not clot as quickly as it used to (clotting agent vitamin K is produced as part of the good bacteria's metabolism), and
- more illness and lower lean muscle mass because of overall lowered immune function.

This often happens especially in situations of high stress, antibiotic use, laxatives and excess heavy metals from the environment, or if you have mercury tooth fillings.

Also, a diet too low in protein intake is another common problem. You need protein to make good intestine linings. However, if you follow the protein guidelines in **(9.3)** you should be fine.

A common solution is to add prebiotics (or soluble fiber), and probiotics, as well as fermented foods such as kimchi, natural yoghurt buttermilk, sauerkraut and miso. As you can see from the above list, most cultures around the world have some kind of traditional fermented food, which was commonly eaten and is good for their digestion.

The dosing recommendation for probiotics comes from one of the best "gut doctors" around, Dr. Suzanne Mack. If you are going to take probiotics, get one from a reputable brand **(9.8)** and take one or two capsules at the end of the day, or two hours after antibiotic use, twice per day.

A diet full of processed trans-fats, as well as refined carbohydrates **(9.1, 9.2)** also encourage bad bacteria growth. So, you would want to stay away from those items to give the good bacteria more chance to grow.

Step 4: Repair damaged structures in your gut.

Once you have put the previous three steps in place, it's time to repair any damage that stress that bad foods and bad habits may have caused. The top nutrients for this are zinc carnosinate, the amino acid glutamine, curcumin and a good quality omega-3 supplement.

4.3 What to look for if you still have problems

Almost certainly, if you follow the steps given above closely, you will have a much better digestive system and overall health. However, as stubborn symptoms remain, the following tests will help you root them out.

Food sensitivity/allergy tests

The best one available is the mediator release test from Signet Diagnostics. It gives the most accurate indicator of what foods cause a bad inflammatory reaction in your body.

The disadvantage is that it is only available in Europe and the USA. This is because the labs that perform this test require blood that is fresh, so long transport times, even by next-day air couriers, are not acceptable.

If the MRT is not available to you, the next best options are immune response tests from Metametrix Lab and ALCAT. In fact, there is even a home kit called "Food Detective" that is fairly accurate, more affordable, and can get you a result within a few hours. Rather than a few weeks as is the period for most labs. Search for providers of these tests in your local area. They should cost approximately $500-600 USD (in 2012 dollars), and $300 USD for the Food Detective.

If a clinic is charging you much more than that, go somewhere else. I believe healthcare practitioners should make their living on their consultation skills, not by marking up lab prices.

For symptomatic relief of symptoms caused by sensitive foods, there is an acupressure technique called NAET (Nambudripad's Allergy Elimination Techniques), which uses acupressure to relieve symptoms of food intolerance. I have had clients who have used this technique with success, and it is especially useful for children with autism.

Stool tests

The next level of tests is for pathogens and good/bad bacteria levels in the gut. These are usually stool tests and the most reputable ones tend to be from Doctors Data Lab. More possible tests you can do are in the lab test section of this book **(10.1)**.

Chapter 5

LIFESTYLE DISEASES

James was a high-level manager in a multinational IT company but over time, he had gained weight and lost health. He had type two diabetes, and was on the maximum dose of cholesterol lowering medication. His weight had increased by more than 40kg to more than 260lbs (about 120kg) and his body fat was close to 40%. The great thing is that James was 100% dedicated to change and he started eating a diet with zero refined carbohydrates, high in omega-3 and natural fat, as well as resistance training three times per week. All of these changes vastly improved his insulin sensitivity and body composition. It was not an easy journey but over nine months he got to a healthy weight (about 83kg), was completely off all medication and was able to complete three triathlons within the following year.

Key Point: dedication to lifestyle changes can make a dramatic effect that is long-lasting

This chapter will describe the shift in "killer diseases" from infectious diseases of the centuries past, to the lifestyle related diseases, which are the common problems faced today. Easy to implement preventive measures to these common lifestyle diseases will be given.

- diabetes,
- cancer, and
- cardiovascular conditions.

5.1 Past and present, what's the difference?

The kinds of illness people get
In the past, the main cause of death was infectious disease because of bacteria, unsanitary living conditions, poor sewage systems and poor medical knowledge in the field of public health. However, according to the latest statistics available in 2012 by the world health organization, thirty-six out of fifty-seven million global deaths were because of non-communicable diseases. These "lifestyle" diseases used to be problems with which only a few rich, sedentary and overfed people had to deal with. Now they are the norm in developed countries.

Medical knowledge and public health systems in developed countries are fairly well equipped to handle infectious disease. However, lifestyle diseases are a totally different ballgame because to be successful against them, there isn't much that laws can do. To win against chronic, lifestyle disease requires consistently good habits and choices by each individual person. Therefore, the battle against them can only be won based on individual accountability and personal responsibility.

The way our food is produced
While this book is not meant to cover the subject of the world's food supply and population growth, there is certainly a difference in the way food is produced today versus as early as a hundred years ago.

In the past, most food was produced on local farms with animals roaming to find feed. However, today, most food is produced on mass farms and by "feed-lots" of caged animals. Most meals also were prepared at home, and almost all food simply looked like food.

It has come to a point where the next generations of children have trouble even recognizing unprocessed food. In an interesting television episode by healthy eating advocate and celebrity chef Jamie Oliver, raw veggies were brought into a classroom of kindergarten kids. Shockingly, the children were not able to identify even basic food items like potatoes and tomatoes. They only recognized processed fast foods like potato chips, and tomato sauce! The conclusion? Children are only likely to eat what they recognize and they don't recognize real food.

If you want to take control of your nutrition, and your health, you will need to understand that several large, for-profit companies currently control much of the world's food supply. The only way they can continue to boost profits, executive bonuses and investor share prices, is to sell more food. That means it is in their interest for us to eat more food, and more of their high-profit, processed food in particular. And to do this, food is made to be as addictive as possible. Unfortunately, it's far easier to entice people to eat more chocolate bars than it is to encourage them to eat more broccoli!

The ill effects of pollution
Something else that affects the entire globe is the amount of chemicals in our environment. In general, industries do not have to prove that chemicals they produce are safe for humans and the environment. Instead it is government and non-profit watchdog organizations who have to prove that chemicals are harmful.

The effects of pollution are so widespread that even newborn babies in "clean" and remote locations like Alaska and Pacific islands, have been found to have chemicals like jet fuel and fire retardants in their blood.

While pollution doesn't instantly kill in most cases, there is a huge variance in each person's ability to deal with it. Some people do well detoxifying petroleum fumes, while others may do well on cigarette smoke. People who are exposed to things they are poor at detoxifying are likely to quickly get ill. For example, those who get sick, or have brain damage from mercury toxicity can have mercury toxicity from an exposure more than one-hundred-twenty days ago; when the average person clears it out in thirty to sixty days.

The stress levels to which we are exposed

Stress is a multi-factorial problem. Poor nutrition and pollution add to our overall stress load. Because of this multitude of factors, it is estimated that our generation is exposed to one-hundred times more overall stress than our grandfather's generations. While they were exposed to more manual labor, the human body is quite well equipped to deal with those kinds of stresses.

Today, we often have pollution, electromagnetic radiation and constant emotional stress from reduced family support, increased job pressures and more job deadlines. These kinds of stresses, we are not well equipped to deal with because they tend to be low grade and not immediately life threatening but rather constant and ongoing. The human body is not so well equipped to deal with this kind of stress.

5.2 Common myths and misconceptions

In my experience, the most common misconception is that there will eventually be a "pill for my ill." This will never happen. There is no way to "fix" a problem with a drug, without transferring the stress to another system in your body.

For example:

- Antibiotics may kill bacteria but they also kill good bacteria in your gut. So, the stress is transferred to your digestive tract.

- Chemotherapy does kill cancer cells but it places a huge burden on your immune system.
- Diabetes medication does lower blood sugar in the short term but it tends to make you fatter in the long-term.
- Cholesterol lowering medication does cut off cholesterol production but it places stress on many systems, including the muscular system, and blood sugar regulation.
- Blood pressure diuretic medication can cause type two diabetes, possible kidney damage and reduces amounts of key nutrients such as potassium and magnesium.
- Beta-blockers (another type of blood pressure medication) can cause impotence, fatigue, lowered good cholesterol, and diabetes.

The list goes on. In general, and if necessary, we should take the smallest doses of any drug, for the shortest time possible. Just remember, drugs don't have side effects. They only have effects!

As you can see, for example, with diuretics and beta blockers, they may lower blood pressure (good) but they also can increase other risk factors of heart disease (bad). So, your overall risk of heart disease may hardly be changed or even increased … totally missing the point!

The key is not to hope for a pill but to build your body's defenses to a high level of excellence so they are ready to fight any potential invader or cancerous cell. To do that, you need optimal levels of nutrients, stress management strategies and exercise.

5.3 Diabetes and metabolic syndrome

Diabetes is a common condition that people have when they start a training program. At Genesis Gym, we probably see at least twenty such cases each year.

I will be talking mostly about type II diabetes because that is almost completely lifestyle related and fixable (i.e. you ate yourself into it!) It is almost impossible to get type II diabetes if you eat low amounts of refined carbohydrates, and have sufficient good protein and healthy fats.

For those who consistently follow the guidelines given below, almost all are able to reduce their blood sugar regulating medication (with the approval of their doctor) within days to weeks, and are off medication totally within about three months on average, depending on their condition when they start.

Also, when talking about type II diabetes, please understand that it is a continuum. You do not wake up one day and suddenly have it. Functional medicine and holistic health practitioner Dr. Mark Hyman likes to call this continuum "diabesity." That means that from the moment you start to put on excess weight, or start to get sedentary, you begin the path toward obesity, and increased diabetes risks. The best time to get off this slippery downward slope is not when you have full-blown diabetes with all of the complications and drastic interventions needed. The best time is with the first pound of excess fat.

Metabolic syndrome

If you want to talk about diabetes, it's also a good idea to know about metabolic syndrome. This is a group of risk factors that dramatically increase the risk of type II diabetes, stroke, heart disease. You have it when you have three out of five of the following. While not a complete risk profile, if you are having trouble with these issues that is already a dangerous sign:

- abdominal obesity,
- triglycerides high,
- low HDL,
- elevated blood pressure, or
- high fasting blood sugar.

5.3.1 Type 1 Diabetes

Type I diabetes is not directly lifestyle related, and it's a disease where your body's immune system attacks your own body (also known as an autoimmune disease) leading to an inability to produce blood sugar lowering hormones on your own. There is no quick fix for this situation but building the body with high levels of nutrients will help manage the disease.

If you do have type I diabetes, the best course of action is to make a consultation with a functional doctor in your area. After doing some laboratory testing, that doctor should be able to make some excellent recommendations for the nutrients and lifestyle that can help you manage the type I diabetes really well. Some examples of how nutrients can help with type I diabetes include:

- Strong research-based links to the amount of vitamin D levels and the occurrence of type one diabetes.
- The better a child's vitamin D levels the less likely they are to get type I diabetes. In addition, the guidelines used to treat type II diabetes will also work for type I to reduce the amount of medication you require.
- The general guidelines for vitamin D about 400 IU per day for a baby, and move up to 2000 IU for a young child. However, as with all things, you need to understand that your body is unique. And each person may vary in their ability to create vitamin D from sunlight, as well as their own individual, unique requirements for vitamin D. Check **(9.10.2)** for more info on vitamin D
- Iodine also is involved in managing type I diabetes, reducing patient's dependence on insulin jabs.
- Get your doctor to consider checks for adrenal function and thyroid function as well because these tests will show you how well your body responds to insulin.

- Also check digestion for leaky gut and other digestive issues **(chapter 4)**, as this is another contributing factor for almost all autoimmune disease.

Note: These tips will also aid anyone with type I diabetes as well

5.3.2 Type II diabetes

I don't like to overcomplicate things. To resolve type II diabetes, use the "turn off the tap" strategy **(1.1)**. Type II diabetes is caused by an inability to handle blood sugar properly. So get away from things that raise blood sugar! That means a low carbohydrate diet for now. Once you are leaner **(2.1)**, have more muscle mass from training and better nutrition **(chapters 9 and 12)**, and are more insulin sensitive **(9.9)**, you can add carbohydrates back in the right quantities and the right types. Every nutrition tip in the nutrition chapter will help accomplish this plan. This is the only long-term, medication free solution.

The basics for handling type II diabetes are listed here.

Step 1: Base your diet 100% on:
- zero refined carbohydrates,
- a lot of healthy fat sources,
- vegetables,
- unprocessed protein sources, and
- nothing else.

Step 2: Eat nutrients that help to rebuild your pancreas (which is overburdened from trying to deal with the excess blood sugar), as well as manage blood sugar:
- fenugreek feed,
- bitter melon,
- gymnema leaf extract,
- cinnamon,
- green tea,

- alpha lipoic acid, and
- vitamin C and E.

Step 3: Do resistance training to build lean mass _(12.2)_.
Yes, there are not many complicated things. Don't be sidetracked by people who ask you to keep doing what you are doing and just "take your medication." Type II diabetes is not caused by a "lack" of medication. It is caused by overburdening the body to the point where it fails to handle blood sugar. Change your lifestyle to avoid damage, and give your body's healing processes a chance to sort the problem out. They are, in almost every case, perfectly able to do so.

5.4 Cancer

Cancer is part of everyone's life. Not just because everyone you or I know has probably lost a friend or relative to this disease, but also because there is the possibility of us forming cancer cells all the time. The question is whether our bodies are able to stop this process before it becomes a real problem. The best time to fight cancer is not when it's detectable, and certainly not when it's late stage. The best time is when the first cancerous cell forms!

The key is not to allow these cancer cells to grow, multiply or spread. The means to do that are:

- a strong immune system,
- a good ability to detoxify cancer causing chemicals and hormones,
- good oxygen supply to cells
- high levels of cancer preventing nutrients, and
- good ability to alkalize your body **(5.4.1)**

The ten top tips shown later will help give you the conditions for stopping cancer cell formation and spread. While there is a genetic component **(9.7)** to cancer, especially prostate, colon and breast cancer, the even more important component is what is known as "epi-genetic." That means it's not just about what you genes are but rather how your genes express themselves.

5.4.1 The Lemon Test

The Lemon test is a good overall test of your body's ability to stay alkaline. You will need:

- 7 strips of pH paper, each about 2 inches (5cm) long.
- One tablespoon of fresh (yes it has to be fresh!) lemon juice, mixed with one tablespoon of water.
- A watch or timer

How to do this test?

1. Mix the lemon juice and water and place it in a cup
2. Make some saliva in your mouth
3. Dip the first piece of pH paper on the saliva in your mouth (just a dip, don't suck on the paper)
4. Immediately compare its color with your pH paper chart – this is your **BASELINE** reading
5. Take a few sips (about 4 sips) to down the entire mixture of water and lemon
6. As soon as all the liquid is swallowed, test pH in your mouth's saliva again
7. For the next 5 minutes, in one minute intervals test your saliva's pH with the other 5 strips.

A good result is an "over-compensation" of your body to the acid solution. That means, the reading after drinking the juice will be more acidic (lower pH) than the baseline, but from then on, there will be a rising trend towards higher pH (more alkaline) numbers. Once you get to the 4th or 5th minute readings, they should be higher than the baseline. This is a good response. If you don't get this response, and your 5th reading is not of a higher pH than your baseline, then take note of that, and focus on eating more plant based nutrients. A good greens drink supplement, and a good electrolyte supplement can help you as well.

5.4.2 How genes work

Think of your genes as a library of books containing information on how to multiply cells. Even if one of the "books" in your library gives a higher chance of your cells becoming cancerous, if you put your entire body in a healthy, well nourished, well detoxified state, it is as if that book never gets "read" by the cell reproduction system, and as such, you never get the cancer.

This is what gene expression is about. Having the "bad genetics" is not the end of the world if you have the right, healthy, environment

As for exactly what to "do" to reduce your cancer risks and even to reverse existing cancer, I take my recommendations from one of my mentors in nutrition, Dr. Rob Rakowski, one of the finest nutrition teachers and practitioners around. His specialty is combining natural and prescription-based solutions for cancer, with an emphasis on lifestyle, and nutrient-based methods. He has excellent success with cancers of all kinds. If I could boil down all I have learned from him in the consultations and seminars I have had with him, here are the top ten things to do.

1. **Stop smoking!**

   Lung cancer is the number one cancer in developed countries. Smoking increases its risk in men by twenty-three times, and thirteen times in women.

   Addiction to smoking is not caused by a lack of nicotine or tar in your lungs! It, like any other addiction is caused by an imbalance of brain chemicals; in this case, the chemical known as dopamine. Low dopamine causes a craving for cigarettes because nicotine increases dopamine. However, there are many natural ways to boost dopamine **(6.2)**.

2. **Stay lean.**

Everyone used to think that fat was just a place where we stored food that our bodies haven't used yet but now we know that this is not the case. Fat cells, especially belly fat cells, have a hormonal function as well, and it's not good news for us. As of our current knowledge, fat cells produce seven different inflammation increasing chemicals called adipocytokines. An environment of increased, chronic inflammation increases cancer risk.

3. **Maximize your levels of plant nutrients.**

Plant nutrients slow, stop or reverse cancer cell activity at every step from cell formation to malignancy. Well-done research by Dr. Bruce Aimes at Berkley shows good evidence that increased consumption of fruits and veggies decreases risk of all kinds of cancer. How does this work? Well, high levels of plant nutrients alkalize the body keeping your pH high.

Plant nutrients also increase oxygen flow to cells because they take up nitrogen from the soil, and this means higher levels of nitrous oxide (NO) in your body, which is a nutrient, required for cardiovascular and brain health.

This is bad news for cancer cells because they are anaerobic (non-oxygen using) and they prefer acidic conditions (low pH). The added benefit of an alkalized body, high in plant nutrients, is that this state increases a body's response to chemotherapy if it ever becomes a necessity.

There is a multitude of beneficial plant nutrients and many are talked about in the nutrition section of this book. The best way to take them is to get a wide variety of them. That means a wide variety of fruits and veggies. The latest recommendation by functional medicine doctors is approximately twelve servings (fist-sized) per day for men, and seven to eight for women. If this amount is not possible, then a good greens drink is a good supplement to add to your routine.

4. **Cut out sugars and refined carbohydrates.**

Cancer cells simply LOVE sugar. When they use sugar, they produce a lot of lactic acid as a waste product. The problem is that this creates an acidic environment around the cancer cells, and then this lactic acid is converted back to glucose in a way that actually depletes your body of energy. The result is both a more acidic body that will break down muscle and bone to balance its acidity out, as well as a higher level of sugar ready for use by the cancer cells, a really vicious cycle, which you can stop by cutting our sugars and all processed carbohydrates.

5. **Beware of environmental toxins and hormonal disruptors.**

While some cancers have genetic linkages (prostate, colon and breast especially), most do not have a strong genetic linkage. What is a stronger factor determining risk is actually exposure to environmental toxins and hormone disruptors because these can alter genes, and even more importantly, they can affect gene expression. An excellent non-profit website that ranks everything from water sources to personal care products to cosmetics and foods in terms of how many toxins they have and which ones you should and should not use is called the "Environmental Working Group" and can be found at EWG.org.

6. **Detox with medical foods.**

For most people the most important thing to detoxify is excessive estrogens because they are excessive in today's environment, and lead to higher risk of prostate and breast cancers.

There are good estrogens and there are bad ones. A good detox program will selectively give your body additional resources to clear out bad estrogens. These resources can be eaten in good amounts through medicinal foods, which are pure, non-allergenic, and have the required potency to give you the right levels of nutrients. There is more on this form of detoxification in **(Chapter 11)**.

7. **Eat organic if possible.**
   Organic foods are often but not always, much more nutritious but they are usually cleaner and more toxin free. From EWG. org, here are the top fifteen foods that are cleanest (not as important to get organic), and the top twelve that are the "dirtiest," which means that you should get organic as often as you can.

Dirty Dozen:
- apples,
- celery,
- bell peppers (red, green, etcetera),
- peaches,
- strawberries,
- nectarines,
- grapes,
- spinach,
- lettuce,
- cucumbers,
- blueberries, and
- potatoes.

Clean Fifteen:
- onions,
- sweet corn,
- pineapples,
- avocado,
- cabbage,
- sweet peas,

- asparagus,
- mangoes,
- eggplant,
- kiwi,
- cantaloupe,
- sweet potatoes,
- grapefruit,
- watermelon, and
- mushrooms.

8. **Manage stress.**

We talk more about the damaging effects of stress in other parts of this book **(7.3)** but with respect to cancer, stress drops immune system function because it prematurely ages and decreases the activity of "natural killer" cells, which are your cancer fighting soldiers.

9. **Minimize radiation exposure.**

Diagnostic radiation like X-rays and CT scans. Instead, thermograms (Infrared thermography) and MRI should be used when possible. If radiation is absolutely needed, take the most shielding that you can, and perform the scans over the smallest possible area of your body. For women, a good radiation-free idea is to do weekly self-breast exams so you get an idea of how your breasts feel at different times in your menstrual cycle and you can react better to any abnormal changes.

10. **Exercise.**

Exercise increases oxygenation to cells, creating a bad environment for cancer. From rat studies, as well as human examples like Lance Armstrong, exercise during cancer treatment prevents the chemo drugs from damaging your heart.

5.4.3 Should I work on smoking first or obesity?

Ideally, you start changing both problems at the same time. However, that much change can be tough to do simultaneously.

There isn't much debate about obesity and smoking being bad for you. For a quick recap, here are some of the bad things about being fat. If you can't see your abs at least a little bit, you are probably on the wrong side of 15% body fat (men) / 22% (women) and need to watch out. This is a non-exhaustive list but there is certainly an increased risk of:

- heart conditions;
- poorer blood profile;
- diabetes;
- stroke;
- sleep apnea;
- hypertension (high blood pressure);
- gout;
- depression; and
- being slow and clumsy, and having poor energy (my unscientific but pretty accurate observation, especially since I too was overweight for a large portion of my childhood, and my team and I help people burn fat for a living).

Smoking has its list of bad consequences as well. It really doesn't matter if it's cigarettes, hookah, or cigars. Although some research indicates that hookah (shisha) may be the worst of the lot.

- Smoking tobacco is instantly addictive, as nicotine is a strong addictive agent.
- If the level of nicotine in a cigarette is condensed into liquid and injected intravenously it will kill you in an instant.
- Tobacco contains close to forty-three carcinogens or cancer inducing agents.

- Nicotine plays havoc with your nerves and works towards hardening them.
- In close to a year of smoking you can contract erectile dysfunction, impotence or soft penile erections.
- Smoking claims the lives of 60% of the smokers through heart disease long before they reach middle age (before the age of forty).
- Smoking is the main cause of asthma in smokers.
- Smoking is not pleasurable but just an addiction, similar to heroin addiction. Cigarettes generate craving for nicotine and the pleasure is just the fulfillment of the nicotine craving in your body.
- Addiction to cigarettes is no different from addiction to cannabis, marijuana, cocaine, heroin or any other drug.
- Tobacco is far more addictive than heroin or marijuana and the addiction is almost instant (after the first cigarette).
- Smoking can cause permanent hardening of arteries and blockage, which are not reversible, leading to heart attack, permanent impotence for life (no more sex), limb atrophy (legs don't receive blood circulation).
- Smoking lights have no advantage over smoking regular cigarettes.
- Tobacco is laced with several other chemicals to make it burn better. The names of these chemicals are no revealed by the manufacturers.
- There are more than 4,000 different chemicals in a cigarette.

Both of these are bad. So which one should I work on first?

In my experience, it is better to work on the obesity and fat loss first. I find that it's a lot easier to work on stopping the smoking later. In fact, sometimes smoking stops on its own.

Every year at Genesis Gym, my team and I have clients come up to us and nonchalantly say *"Oh, by the way, I just quit smoking."* Why does this happen? To find out, we need to look at some of the reasons people smoke.

- Smoking is pleasant and relaxing (helps with anger stress, anxiety, sadness, etcetera).
- Smoking helps relieve boredom.

When a person is depressed, or bored, it usually means a lower level of the brain chemicals dopamine and acetylcholine. These chemicals are likely to be returned to normal when a person loses fat in a healthy way. Some of the factors that are in any safe and effective fat loss program are:

- exercise in a positive environment,
- good social support,
- a nutritious diet of unprocessed food, and
- supplements to restore nutrient levels.

These activities and nutrients boost natural levels of dopamine and acetylcholine **(5.2)**, which means fewer cravings for smoking. Meat, nuts and a low glycemic/low insulin diet tend to burn fat and increase the levels of these brain chemicals. That's why if you have both a need to smoke and kilos to lose, you should work on the kilos first and then surprise yourself when quitting the smokes becomes easier, too.

5.5 Cardiovascular conditions (heart disease and hypertension)

Cardiovascular conditions are the number one killer worldwide and statistics from the World Health Organization suggest that heart-related conditions claim 29% of the people who die each year.

The person I turn to for heart and cardiovascular condition advice is Dr. Mark Houston, who was recently voted one of the one-hundred most influential doctors in America, and runs probably the best natural medicine, cardiovascular health clinic you can find anywhere in Nashville, Tennessee.

5.5.1 What are the "traditional" markers of heart health?

Usually, the indicators that most physicians examine to determine heart disease risk are:

- cholesterol levels—trying to be below two-hundred mg/dL;
- LDL levels—try to be below 100mg/dL;
- high blood pressure—depending on the lab, somewhere below 130/80;
- diabetes—usually checked with fasting blood glucose below 110mg/dL;
- obesity—using BMI **(2.3)**; and
- smoking.

However, these readings do not give a complete picture, because they do not relate very closely to actual cardiovascular disease risk. Now we know that it is actually inflammation, oxidative stress and autoimmune damage that are the key causes of problems for cardiovascular health because of the damage they cause to the linings of your blood vessels. In addition, there is a genetic factor involved with cardiovascular risk as well.

At present, there are more than seven-hundred known gene locations where errors can increase cardiovascular risk. However, as you will see in **(5.4.1)** you can overcome much of the genetic variances with a good lifestyle. By working on the conditions listed in this chapter, you will certainly reduce your risk of cardiovascular conditions.

5.5.2 Inflammation

Inflammation is normal, and actually is designed to prevent infection because inflammation triggers a response by your immune system. In the short term, it is a great defense mechanism but in the longer term the "attack mode" of your immune system can damage your own cells. This form of chronic inflammation is bad for all kinds of diseases including diabetes and cancer as well.

The most common indicator of high inflammation that you can find in a regular health check is called HS-CRP (or sometimes just CRP). This is a substance released by your liver when the body is in an inflammatory state. A good reading is under 2.0mg/L.

Common things that increase inflammation:
- refined carbohydrates,
- trans-fats,
- smoking,
- poor sleep quality,
- lack of physical activity, and
- infectious diseases.

What do you do about it?
There are many nutrients that are well researched to lower inflammation but if you tried to take a few capsules of each of these in supplement form each day you would be taking in fifty or more capsules per day … not particularly convenient (information from Houston HD book, page 34/277).

So, I will give you some "best bang for the buck" solutions here that should help almost everyone lower inflammation to a healthy status. If not, then you can consider taking some of the other items on the list, and go for more comprehensive laboratory testing **(Chapter 10)** to see what other things might help you.

- Diet should be anti-inflammatory—healthy fats, fruits and veggies, low refined carbohydrates **(Chapter 9)**.
- Exercise—Drops some inflammation markers (Hs-CRP) by up to 50% in studies. Other studies show that resistance training drops it by 32.8% and cardio by 16.1% so if you are pressed

for time, strength training is certainly a better bet. An excellent strength training workout is available in **(Chapter 12)**.

- Omega-3 supplements—Many studies showing lowered inflammation markers with omega-3 especially the EPA component of omega-3.
- GLA—boosts your body's own anti-inflammatory compounds and it works great together with omega-3s.
- Vitamin C and E—these are powerful antioxidants of the cardiovascular system.

5.5.3 Oxidative stress and free radical damage

Oxygen is a necessity for life but part of the reaction that creates energy in our cells also creates molecules called "free radicals." These free radicals usually are not a problem because your body has a built in system of "antioxidants," which can usually calm down these very reactive free radicals.

The problems begin to happen when you produce too many free radicals for the antioxidants to fix, or you have too few or the wrong kinds of antioxidants. Extra free radicals are bad news because they attack other molecules and will steal an electron from them to balance themselves out. This leaves the victim lacking electrons and now the new atom goes in search of another victim from which to steal electrons.

If this vicious cycle goes on for too long, it leaves a wake of unbalanced, damaged molecules which cannot perform their duties well, and that means damaged tissues, organs and cells mutation. Some of the conditions that are caused by, and or sped up by free radical damage include:

- aging,
- Alzheimer's,
- arthritis,
- atherosclerosis,
- cancer,

- cataracts,
- diabetes,
- heart attack,
- Multiple Sclerosis,
- Parkinson's Disease
- stroke.

Almost all chronic diseases have a free-radical component.

Naturally, the way to beat free radicals is to produce as few of them as we can, and to protect ourselves with as many antioxidants as we can. Here are some sources of antioxidants. Internally produced antioxidants—alpha lipoic acid, CoQ10, glutathione, melatonin.

Twenty best food sources according to the USDA:

- red beans,
- wild blueberries,
- kidney beans,
- pinto beans,
- farm-raised blue berries,
- cranberries,
- artichokes,
- blackberries,
- prunes,
- raspberries,
- strawberries,
- Red Delicious apples,
- Granny Smith apples,
- pecans,
- cherries,
- black plums,
- russet potato,
- black beans,

- plums, and
- Gala apples.

Other sources

- whey protein,
- green tea,
- resveratrol (from wines),
- curcumin (active ingredient in turmeric),
- flavaniods (from coffee, fruits, veggies etcetera),
- zinc (meat, eggs, seafood),
- selenium (brazil nuts, meat, fish),
- vitamin C (fruits and vegetables),
- vitamin E (vegetables and beans),
- reduced form Alpha Lipoic Acid, and
- N-Acetyl-Cystine.

This is a long (and yet still incomplete) list. However, as you can see there is a wide variety of sources of antioxidants. This is because there is no single, best, magic antioxidant **(1.4)**. Antioxidants differ in the areas in which they "specialize." For example, vitamin E is excellent for protection of reproductive organs in women and in preventing oxidation of unsaturated fats, and zinc is excellent for protection of the eyes. In addition, antioxidants need to "recycle" each other because they are "one shot" wonders. Once an antioxidant has neutralized a free radical, it needs to be recycled by other antioxidants before it can be used again.

So what should a basic antioxidant-rich lifestyle look like?
- diet—Omega-3s, mono unsaturated fats, fruits/veggies/low refined carbs;
- exercise;
- Coq10;

- green tea (EGCG);
- resveratrol; and
- vitamin C and E.

As you can see, an antioxidant-rich diet is very similar to an anti-inflammatory diet **(5.5.2)**. For supplements, a broad-based antioxidant formula, along with a greens drink should cover your bases if you are not getting enough variety or quantity of fruits and veggies in your daily diet.

5.5.4 Emotional stress

Emotional stresses increase free radical production. This is because of the stress hormones you make breaking down into free radicals. Stress management methods from prayer, light stretching, soothing music and a grateful log **(See 3.3 for more on stress)** can go a long way to defusing dangerous stress hormones. In short—for oxidative stress of all kinds—take in antioxidants, exercise and manage stress.

5.5.5 What about cholesterol?

Cholesterol is probably the best-known risk factor for heart disease, even if it's not the most important one. This incorrect idea in no small part is because cholesterol-lowering medication is well marketed by the billion dollar per year pharmaceutical industry.

The other factors related to heart disease are reduced by lifestyle and nutritional changes. If people took this route, there would be fewer patients and not much money to be made. So these methods are less well known.

Cholesterol ranges in laboratory tests are also a problem. Most laboratory tests simply say that a good range is "lower than two-hundred (or two-hundred-twenty-five depending on lab)." So is zero good? Certainly not. Cholesterol is necessary for healthy muscle, digestion and hormone function so even though zero is within the "acceptable" lab range, you will be dead! In addition, before the arrival of cholesterol lowering drugs, the normal range of total cholesterol was 180 to 340 mg/dl, far higher than todays' norms, and yet people had less heart disease.

The two most well-known types of cholesterol are HDL and LDL, with HDL being "good" and LDL being "bad." However, this is not an accurate representation of what's actually going on. There are at least five different kinds of HDL. Some are small and dense, and some are large and fluffy. The small and dense ones (called HDL-3) are not protective, while the fluffy big ones (called HDL-2 and HDL-2B) are protective. There are at least five types and sizes of LDL as well but they are all "lumped" together when you get a cholesterol report. Like HDL, they range from small and dense to large and fluffy.

The small and dense ones are the most damaging because they can be stuck in the walls of your arteries and are more easily oxidized and glycated (corrupted by a sticky sugar-like substance), which leads to inflammation and artery hardening, as well as a greater risk of stroke and heart attacks. It's these "problem" type cholesterols that are much more damaging than the actual total amount of cholesterol that you have, (which is what all the most common tests measure).

It's true that most check-ups will not contain this information. But that's okay, what's most important is what you can do to improve your cholesterol profile from what it is now, to what it should be for maximum health. What you want is HDL and LDL that is big and fluffy so they never get stuck and damage you.

To get big fluffy, healthy cholesterol molecules, you want to:

- stop smoking;
- stop eating refined carbohydrates;
- stop eating trans-fats **(9.2);**
- exercise;
- maintain a healthy weight and body fat level; and
- increase intake of anti-inflammatory nutrients such as omega-3, pantathine, niacin, plant sterols, vitamin E and

green tea, which (lowers bad types of LDL, raises good types of HDL, and most importantly, reduces oxidation of LDL).

Some good test results are:

- LDL total <900 per mg/DL,
- Lipoprotein a < thirtymg/dl,
- Triglycerides <75 mg/DL,
- VLDLD <75mg/DL, and
- HDL min 40-50, ideal >80mg/dl.

5.5.6 Blood pressure

Medicines can help but there are side effects **(5.2)**. So, we only use them when necessary, only once we have found out exactly what the cause of the blood pressure problem is, and once natural alternatives have proven to be ineffective.

What is blood pressure?

Blood pressure is a combination measure of the "pump" of your heart, and the ability of your arteries, to relax and accommodate the blood coming from your heart. Arteries are muscles too! So, if either the heart, or the arteries have problems, blood pressure can rise.

How is it read?

BP readings are shown as a "fraction" with one number above another. These two numbers represent two different times of measurement. The top, larger number is the pressure when the heart is beating (also called systolic pressure). The lower, smaller number is the pressure when the heart relaxes (also known as diastolic pressure). The difference between the two numbers is called the pulse pressure.

How to test blood pressure correctly.

Blood pressure is a sensitive measurement. Small changes in the conditions of the test can give significant differences in the measurement. For example, my brother who is a very healthy guy, exercises four to five times per week, and is very lean, has had a "dangerously high" blood pressure when he went for his company's pre-employment health check. This was no surprise to me after he described the rush that patients were put in to have all of their health checks done. This increase in activity and stress levels is almost certain to give a higher than normal blood pressure reading.

- No matter if you are reading your blood pressure at home or in a clinical setting, here are some guidelines that will help you get an accurate and consistent reading.
- Don't exercise or move too much for sixty minutes before the measurement
- Don't eat or drink anything for thirty minutes before the measurement
- Don't take any stimulants or medication.
- Complete rest at least five minutes before the measurement. Try to relax; the doctor's office can be a hectic place and can lead to false high readings called "white coat hypertension."
- Try to be in the measurement room early if you can, so that you are adjusted to the surroundings and temperature.
- Take the reading in the morning. Most people have higher readings later in the day because of body rhythm.
- Make sure your clothing is loose and that your sleeve does not restrict your arm in any way.
- Make sure that your elbow is at heart level, any lower and pressure goes up significantly.

- Make sure that the blood pressure cuff is the right size. If you are especially large or small, ask the doctor for a suitable size cuff.
- Ideally, take readings on both arms.

Phew! That's a long list. In reality, most medical practitioners know about these items. However, it is your responsibility as a patient to know them as well, to make sure that no steps are missed and that you get the best possible reading. Don't feel bad if you ask the nurse or doctor to do a remeasurement if you believe any of the above list was not in order.

What is good/bad blood pressure?

- High pulse pressure. Remember, that's the difference between top and bottom numbers, is bad. Anything more than forty is dangerous. It means your arteries are stiff and unable to relax to handle the pumping of blood.
- No dip at night. You should have about a 10% drop in blood pressure at night. Any more or less than this is not a good sign.
- Excessive increase in the morning. 5% up is normal, anything more than 20% is not good.
- Poor blood pressure response to exercise. Usually, blood pressure should not consistently go over 180 systolic (the top number) and not much change on diastolic (the bottom number). If systolic is higher than that, or diastolic rises, they are bad signs.

Why is high blood pressure bad?

High-pressure blood hits arteries harder causing damage just like a fast-moving river wears down its banks. When this happens, there is increased inflammation, oxidative stress and autoimmune dysfunction **(5.5.2, 5.5.3)**. Your kidneys also take a greater burden and most importantly, the sensitive endothelium of your arteries gets damaged, which makes all other factors worse.

What causes it to rise?
- caffeine is a common cause especially for those who do not detoxify it well. A good indicator if you are one of these people is if you have trouble relaxing even many hours after a cup of coffee;
- low levels of vitamins C, D, E, magnesium, coq10;
- high levels of stress hormones, trans-fats, uric acid;
- smoking; and
- obesity, each pound of fat is a mile more blood vessels for your heart to pump blood through

What can you do about it?
Eat well known natural blood pressure lowering nutrients and foods. It's important to get a variety. In many cases, overdosing one single nutrient is not ideal; rather, it's the combination that gives a better effect. It is much harder to get a 20% improvement from a single nutrient than it is to get a 3% improvement from many nutrients:

- dark chocolate;
- CoQ10—also is an antioxidant, and falls after age thirty;
- plant nutrients and flavonoids—found in fruit and veggies, wine, coffee, teas;
- garlic—lowers blood pressure, inflammation, and oxidative stress;
- hawthorn—is anti-inflammatory and reduces oxidative stress;
- lycoprene—increases the quality of your blood vessel lining;
- Melatonin—is anti-inflammatory and reduces oxidative stress;
- omega-3;
- vitamin K—counteracts salt for those who are sensitive to salt;

- vitamin C—for ability of arteries to relax/contract, antioxidant properties;
- vitamin D—regulates BP; and
- whey—lowers BP, has ingredients that help produce antioxidants

In general—diet, exercise, supplements: the top three are dark chocolate (75% or more) 30g, coQ10 100mg and vitamin C 500mg.

5.5.7 Blood sugar

More sugar = lower HDL, more triglycerides, insulin resistance, elevated blood sugar, inflammation, oxidative stress, autoimmune damage in arteries and thus, more arterial damage.

The test: A good fasting blood sugar level is 80mg/dl, after that every 1mg increase is 1% risk increase. Because the "normal" range at most laboratories starts from 100mg/dl, that is actually an already increased risk of 20%.

What increases blood sugar?

- refined carbohydrates,
- high fructose corn syrup,
- low Vitamin D,
- low nutrients and electrolytes,
- obesity,
- insulin resistance,
- low lean mass,
- low test, and
- no exercise.

What nutrients lower blood sugar?

- chromium;
- green tea;

- sesamin;
- fiber;
- cinnamon;
- fenugreek;
- bitter melon;
- potassium and magnesium—They help to convert blood sugar into glycogen and control blood sugar and blood pressure. Good sources of potassium are: figs, Papaya, dates, banana. Good sources of magnesium are avocado, almonds, and spinach; and
- most importantly—cut out refined carbohydrates. All of the supplements or nutrients in the world will not be able to help you lower blood sugar if your diet has a lot of processed starches or sugars in it. Stick with the level 1 and 2 carbohydrates in **(9.3.2)**.

In conclusion, when it comes to cardiovascular problems it seems best that we take a "big picture" approach where we look at every factor that can contribute to the problem. The good news is that the solutions cover many of the factors and will reduce them as a group.

Nutrients that lower blood sugar also tend to have antioxidant properties; a diet that helps with blood pressure also is likely to reduce the risk of autoimmune conditions and so on. Following the nutrition guidelines in **(Chapter 9)** and the specialized supplement suggestions shown in this chapter is a great way to keep your cardiovascular system in great working shape.

5.5.8 Lab results? A quick summary

Now that we know that total cholesterol and total LDL are not the most reliable predictors of heart disease, what really does give an indicator of heart disease risk? Here is a summary of some norms for items that are common in most lab tests. If I had to choose the number one risk factor out of all those listed, it would probably be TG/HDL ratio. It is not only indicative of heart disease risk but also of insulin resistance, higher body fat, poorer waist to hip ratio, and higher blood pressure. If you are in the risk zones, it is time to take action.

Risk Factor	Ideal	Moderate Risk	Serious Risk
C-Reactive Protein	<1	>2	>3
Fasting Glucose	87	>100	>110
Fibrinogen	<235	>235	>350
Homocystine	8	>8	>12
Lipoprotein(a) mg/dl	<20	>25	>30
HDL (men)	>60	<50	<40
HDL (women)	>70	<60	<50
Triglycerides (TG)	<100	>100	>150
TG:HDL ratio	1:1	2:1	4:1
VLDL	<20	>30	>40

Chapter 6

Brain function

Steven operates a consulting business and formerly was a national level athlete. However, as he entered his mid to late thirties he found he was not able to focus, concentrate or think as efficiently as before. I suspected that because of his hectic lifestyle, with irregular meals and constant stress, a nutrient-based solution would work well. With high doses of brain friendly omega-3 fats, as well as other nutrients such as huperzine and acetyl-l-carnitine, he reports far greater levels of energy, and the ability to focus and think for hours on end without the need for stimulants of any kind.

Key point: Your brain is an extremely sensitive organ and a malnourished brain is a slow brain!

This chapter links brain function and mood to the body. It will help the reader understand how the brain does not work in isolation but rather as part of the whole body. As such, brain "problems" need to be addressed in a system-wide approach. The main topics covered will include:

- concentration,
- learning and memory,
- mood, and
- long-term brain health.

I have a very strong interest in biochemistry and how our bodies work as a whole system. It is quite clear that habits, food and lifestyle can influence your biochemistry, which directly influences your brain function. If poorly fed, with a diet full of refined sugars and processed foods that increase oxidative stress, glycation and upset brain chemical balance, you will have yet another obstacle to optimum mood, relaxation, drive and focus.

In contrast, when your brain is well nourished, you will have the biochemistry to give a greater boost of motivation, focus and energy while giving you less self-sabotaging and negative thoughts. These will help you reach your goals in other areas of life as well.

Just like any other system in your body, your brain does not work in isolation. It is affected and affects just about every other system. What is special about a brain is that it needs protection because it is probably the most sensitive organ we have. Not just the physical protection that our skull provides but also protection from toxins, nutrient deficiencies and stress.

Our brains weigh roughly 2% of our total body weight but use about 20% of our energy for its incredible processing functions, which the scientific community is only now, just scratching the surface. Giving our brains the nutrients they need for energy and repair can quickly make a big difference in terms in concentration, memory, mood and long-term brain health, with a far lower risk of brain-related illness.

6.1 Brain health basics

Step 1

The first thing you need to do for brain health is to lower insulin levels. Insulin is the only hormone we have complete control over because it is determined by how much, and what types of food we eat. Consistently high insulin levels over time age the brain and damage it. The risk of Alzheimer's disease, which was voted in a Metlife foundation's survey as one of the "scariest" diseases to get in old age, is actually greatly reduced by making sure we keep insulin in check.

High insulin from refined carbohydrates also tends to lead to a spike in stress hormones two to three hours after the insulin spike. Stress hormones also have a damaging effect on the brain, and especially on short-term memory. Following the nutrition guidelines **(Chapter 9)** will drop your insulin to healthy levels.

Step 2

The second thing you need to do for ideal brain health is to fix your digestive tract or gut. The brain and digestive tract are closely linked. Two thirds of your brain chemicals (neurotransmitters) are produced in the gut **(6.2)**.

In fact, it has been estimated that our gut has the additional processing capacity about equal to that of a cat brain. A healthy gut makes sure that this additional capacity is available to us.

The steps to fix your gut in **(4.2, 4.3)** would go a long way to improving and optimizing brain function, since any inflammation, excess bad bacteria and damage to gut lining will affect neurotransmitter levels.

In addition, be aware that gluten from wheat-based products such as bread and pasta can cause damage to the communication system between brain cells.

Step 3

The third thing to do is to manage stress and exercise your brain. Stress management is well covered in the chapter on sleep **(3.1)**. In addition to managing stress, it is important to "exercise" your brain to keep the learning and memory pathways in your brain strong.

The best way to do this is to expose your brain to different kinds of stimuli, varied learning and creative thinking. The people who have lower risks of brain damage tend to be those who have to use their brains daily (e.g., people like athletes who do sports with high levels of coordination required such as martial arts, or gymnastics, as well as those who do mentally challenging jobs like judges or doctors). It doesn't really matter what job you do but it's best to keep learning, challenging yourself and trying to improve yourself in varied ways.

Step 4

The final step is to make sure that your brain is well nourished. The most well researched brain nutrient, with the best bang for the buck, is omega-3 from a good quality fish oil. In particular, the oils that have high levels of DHA.

After that, the second best brain nutrient, which has worked very well in my experience, is what is known as Acetyl-L-Carnitine. This is a focus booster and brain-energizing nutrient that works really well with omega-3s. This is a different nutrient from regular carnitine because the acetyl version is able to cross from your blood into your brain tissues, which the regular carnitine is not able to do. An excellent resource on the benefits of carnitine can be found in *The Carnitine Miracle* by renowned nutritionist Robert Crayhon.

The next two nutrients also work well once your omega-3 and carnitine levels are good. One is alpha glycerylphosphorylcholine (Alpha GPC), which is an excellent booster of acetylcholine, the brain chemical for memory. It also increases the speed at which your nerves conduct signals so you get stronger too! Phosphytidyl Serine (PS) has shown an ability to lower stress, as well as repair the hippocampus, which is the area in your brain responsible for memory.

The documented effects of PS are:

- improved memory,
- reduced effects of aging on your brain,
- prevention of Alzheimer's and other brain-related issues,
- improved conditions of people with depression,
- improved sleep, and
- reduced release of excess stress hormones such as cortisol in response to stressful situations.

Finally, some herb-based nutrients are very effective as well. The two main ones that I have used with success are huperzine (Chinese moss) and ashwaganda.

The benefit of huperzine is that it prevents the breakdown of the memory brain chemical acetylcholine so it lasts longer; thus, your memory improves. The benefit of ashwaganda is that it helps manage stress levels (if needed) and improves energy (if needed). Because of its ability to do both of these things, herbs such as ashwaganda are called "adaptogenic."

6.2 Brain chemicals (neurotransmitters)

6.2.1 Neurotransmitter basics

There are four main neurotransmitters (NT). Two of them are more "energizing" and two of them are more "relaxing" but each is different in subtle ways that the Braverman test will help you find. Here are the basics of brain chemistry for you to have a better understanding of your test results.

The key to brain health is not the actual amounts of NT because they are neither good nor bad but rather the balance between them. Balancing your NTs is like having a chair with four legs. The length of each leg is far less important than the fact the four legs are of equal length.

Dopamine and acetylcholine are the two energizing neurotransmitters. They help you have concentration, focus, motivation and better memory. While GABA and serotonin are the relaxing neurotransmitters. They help us relax, de-stress and recover from hard training.

Dopamine is the NT of motivation and drive. It also improves growth hormone output and sex hormone output. So, low dopamine would mean poorer fat burning, and lowered sex drive (or drive for anything actually). It's also linked to addictive habits. Because dopamine is linked to pleasure, if it is low it makes a person more likely to fall victim to "quick fix" sources of pleasure such as food or nicotine. This is why I suggest that clients work on obesity before nicotine addiction **(4.4.1)**.

Acetylcholine is the NT that aids your memory, reaction time and muscle function. Therefore, if you are doing brain intensive work at your job or have an occupation like a police officer or athlete, having optimal acetylcholine is a good idea. The meat and nuts breakfast will help acetylcholine levels. **(9.6.5)**.

GABA (gamma-aminobutyric acid) is the NT that helps a person deal with anxiety. This is a commonly deficient NT and my own Braverman test even indicates this in me. You can think of GABA as the "opposite" of dopamine. It is well and good to be driven and motivated (good dopamine levels) but if you can't relax and recover at the end of each day (low GABA) you will eventually wear yourself out.

Serotonin is the NT that counters depression. Low levels make a person feel depressed, disconnected and "tired of life." Good levels make a person feel confident and vibrant. Serotonin deficiency tends to express itself in the typical depression symptom of feeling "numb." Different from GABA deficiency, which makes a person feel anxious or worried. Sleeping better will certainly improve serotonin levels **(Chapter 3)**.

6.2.2 The Braverman Test

One additional test that I help clients do to customize their brain nutrition further is called the "Braverman" test designed by Dr. Eric Braverman and described in his book, *The Edge Effect*.

Dr. Braverman is one of the top experts on brain health and neurotransmitter balance. This test is a check to see in which of the four brain chemicals (neurotransmitters) you are dominant, and in which you are deficient.

There is no right or wrong to the tests. However, there are indicators that you can feed yourself certain foods and nutrients that can help your brain function optimally. Your scores will also show the severity of the dominance and deficiency and the food and nutrient recommendations will need to be adjusted accordingly.

After getting the results of this test, you will have two scores. One score for the brain chemical in which you are most dominant, and one in which you are most deficient. Primarily, you will need to focus on nutrients that help replenish your deficiency but you will also benefit from some nutrients (in lower doses) that fuel your dominance. These nutrients are also described in his book.

If you feel that your habits and lifestyle are already excellent, but neurotransmitter imbalance is still a road-block for you, Dr. Bravermans' book is an excellent resource and you should consider doing the test. It is Q & A based and should take you about 30 minutes to complete.

Chapter 7

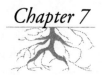

Aging

This chapter will cover the main causes of aging. This is the shortest chapter in the book because, while aging is an important topic, our body is so interconnected that the main causes are all covered pretty well in other chapters. To avoid repetition, I will put the links in here for your reference.

7.1 The main causes of premature aging are:

Excessive inflammation. To work on this, improve your:

- sleep (Chapter 3),
- digestive health (Chapter 4),
- food quality (Chapter 9), and
- chronic injury issues (Chapter 8).

Excessive stress. Work on your:

- sleep (Chapter 3), and
- digestive health (Chapter 4).

Excessive glycation. Work on your nutrition:

- details about glycation (Chapter 9.3.3).

Excessive oxidative damage. Make sure your defenses are in order:

- nutrition and supplementation (Chapter 9.8),
- lab testing (chapter 10.5), and
- cardiovascular health (chapter 5.5).

Chapter 8

CHRONIC PAIN

Grace is a mother of two young kids. Since having her second child, she had been having nagging back pain. On our initial assessment, it was found that her quadratus lumborum muscles, which stabilize one side of her hips, along with her multifidus muscles, which stabilize her spine, were not functioning correctly. She also had scar tissue in her lower back from an old dancing injury.

The correct choice for treatment of the muscle dysfunction was the "trigenincs" method of muscle strengthening, and the correct choice for the scar tissue was acupuncture needles along with a soft tissue treatment technique to break up the scar tissue. The needles and the soft tissue treatment allowed oxygen to flow in the scared area again. Just two treatments later, she was pain free, and a good strength-training program makes it very unlikely that the pain will occur again.

Key Point: Stay strong to prevent injury, and choose the right treatment for the right kind of problem.

This chapter will cover the main pain-related issues that are common in many people's lives. Body part by body part, it will cover the common aches and strains found in many people. It will also cover the relationship between pain, nutrition and other body systems, as well as the relationship between pain in different parts of the body and how one injury can lead to another.

It will also have multiple illustrations of common exercises, stretches and treatments that help relieve pain and will include a section about finding a good therapist in your area who can help your needs.

8.1 Main cause of chronic pain

Chronic pain can come from many sources including old injuries, bad sleeping or posture habits, improper carrying of objects, tumors, organ related pain, bones and nerves, or even exercise done with the wrong technique or in excessive amounts.

The main source of long-term chronic pain comes from the musculo-skeletal system. That means the taking care of your muscles and connective tissue can usually help you make great improvements in your levels of chronic pain.

8.2 Different treatment options

There are several methods, that when used at the right time, can be almost magical in relieving chronic pain. The methods listed here are not exhaustive but they are the ones that I either use as a practitioner, or have referred clients to with consistently positive results. According to Olympic coach Ian King, one of the keys to long-term health is to balance out "tension producing" and "tension reducing" activities. Training and overall stress **(3.3)** on your body is tension producing. While almost all the treatment methods listed below are tension reducing. Ideally, for every hour of training you do, or for every hour you spend exercising, sitting, standing or lying in a position of bad posture, you should spend an equal time in a lengthened position to balance out the tension.

Stretching

Multiple methods of stretching are out there. The ones that I like most are fascial stretching, and PNF stretching. There also is benefit to light (not full tension) stretching held for longer periods up to twenty minutes or more because these long stretches can help teach your nervous system that the new, more flexible position is normal, thus, keeping the benefits long-term.

Pros:
- The biggest and most important benefit of stretching is that, when done well, it has the longest lasting effect on flexibility of any method. It also is free and many excellent stretches can be done alone, free, with minimal or no equipment.

Cons:
- Effects take a while to take hold. You need to be committed to doing stretching for a significant time (about thirty minutes or more per day) for a long period (at least eight weeks)
- There can be confusion about when and what kind of stretching to use at different times of the day.
- Some parts of your body like your illiotibial (IT) band do not respond well to stretching. They require other forms of treatment like ART, or massage.

My favorite stretching book is *Stretch to Win* by Ann and Chris Fredericks. Ideally, it's best to take a session with one of their fascial stretch therapists (www.stretchtowin.com) to get an idea of how the technique works in person.

Foam rolling/self-massage tools/trigger point therapy

These can be firm balls, rollers and other tools that provide pressure similar to human fingers. Alternatively, they can be done with fingers and hands of a therapist. They work by several mechanisms but one of the major ones is stopping blood flow temporarily with their pressure, then allowing an excess flow of blood to rush into the affected area when the pressure is released.

Pros:
- affordable, effective for trigger point pain,
- simple, can be done at home with simple equipment, and
- can usually feel benefits within days.

Cons:
- takes a bit of skill to use correctly,
- does not address scar tissue or brain-muscle connection effectively, and
- may not be solving root cause of problem, does not adequately address brain-muscle connection.

Good basic resource:
Trigger Point Therapy Workbook, Claire Davies.

Active Release Technique (ART)

This is an excellent treatment technique that breaks up scar tissue and "stuck" areas of soft tissue by a combination of tension and pressure from the therapists' hands, and movement by the patient's body.

Pros:
- for scar tissues, it is absolutely amazing with nearly instant results;
- pain relief and range of motion increase is instantaneous; and
- long lasting results as long as you don't reinjure yourself.

Cons:
- requires a skilled practitioner,
- not all practitioners are of equal ability despite equal qualifications, and
- does not address brain-muscle connection directly.

To find a practitioner in your area, visit www.activerelase.com.

Biomedical Dry Needling

This western method of pain management and injury treatment uses acupuncture needles to affect muscles, nerves and connective tissue by increasing blood-flow and tissue quality.

Pros:
- able to reach "inside" the body effectively to target deep muscles, scar tissue and connective tissue that fingers or tools cannot reach; and
- fast results because needles have a "whole body" positive effect even when targeted at only a specific area.

Cons:
- requires a skilled practitioner.
- There may be a "fear-factor" when dealing with needles – but in reality, the discomfort that bad, it is more of a "weird" feeling of something under your skin, rather than a sharp pain.

Trigenics

Trigenics is a technique that works well because the patient is involved heavily in the treatment. The therapist provides tension while the patient combines movement with relaxation breathing. This combination "resets" the muscle-brain connection and restores correct muscle length and strength.

Pros:

- instant pain relief and strength boosting,
- addresses brain-muscle connection.

Cons:

- requires a skilled practitioner,
- does not address scar tissue so will need a combination with other treatment if scar tissue is part of the problem.

Frequency specific micro-current (FSM)

FSM uses two channels of low power electric current to instruct different tissues to heal. One channel is a frequency that tells the body which tissues to "turn on" (e.g., muscle, nerve, organ), and the other channel tells that specific tissue what do to (e.g. repair, reduce inflammation, relax).

Pros:

- can be used all of the time because of convenience of the device,
- one machine has multiple uses from helping with sleep issues to chronic pain to acute injury and reducing inflammation.

Cons:

- best used when "rented" out for long but subtle treatment; "one off" sessions don't work as well in my experience;
- machine is relatively expensive to buy at a personal level (several thousand USD).

Fascial abrasion tool (FAT)

This tool has a grippy surface that helps to shake free scar tissue and connective tissue that is stuck and not moving freely.

Pros:

- excellent for increasing range of motion and releasing scar tissue,
- great for post exercise recovery,
- pain free,
- some parts of your body can be done by yourself so self-treatment is possible, and
- almost impossible to cause harm even with incorrect treatment technique.

Cons:

- some patients may still require ART or similar soft tissue treatment even after FAT tool use

Chiropractic adjustment

This is a well-known treatment method and uses various techniques to put bones and other structures into correct alignment.

Pros:

- one of the only ways to put bony structures back into place, and
- works instantly.

Cons:

- does not "hold" long-term if other issues are the cause of the misalignment.

Note: good chiropractors almost always use a combination with some of the other methods listed above to give better long-term results.

8.3 How to choose the right treatment for your problem

Most people have been injured or have some chronic pain at some time in their life. If you have been one of these people, you will know that it can be frustrating to find the cause of the pain and the solution to the pain. Here is where finding a professional can help you.

The problem is who, where and how do you know this treatment, which will cost you time and money, is going to make things better for you? Here are some guidelines that I use when referring clients out for specialized treatment by other healthcare professionals.

1.   **Stay away from "big packages."**
     A good therapist requires relatively few treatments to give you a benefit. In fact, for most injuries one or two treatments should give you significant improvement. Unless your injury is chronic, AND you are unhealthy (e.g., a lot of tenderness all over your body, no exercise, bad diet) treatments done right should have a significant benefit.

     Therefore, if a place asks you to buy a "package of thirty treatments" then run away quickly. They usually are in it for the money, and not to help you quickly. After all, if you get well fast, you don't need to come back.

2.   **Ask for testimonials.**
     All of the best therapists I know from around the world have testimonials from satisfied clients who got great results. You need to ask for testimonials from people who have a similar condition to yours.

3.   **Make sure they prepare you for treatment.**
     Good therapists do a great job of preparing your body for treatment. They do one or more of the following so that your nervous system and soft tissues are ready to be treated:

- acupuncture,
- frequency specific micro-current,
- massage,
- infrared lamp, and
- some kind of gentle stretching.

They also ask the right questions, and observe the right things to find the root causes of your problem. A good therapist should include a health and injury history and some form of muscle or movement testing.

These are the guys who care. Those who only want as many patients and profit as possible and don't care as much about results, ask you to lie down, crack your bones left and right and say "thank you, see you next week."

4. **Use the right method for your problem.**

Injury treatment is a little like martial arts. Sometimes it is best to use punches, sometimes elbows, sometimes kicks and sometimes wrestling. Similarly, your problem needs the right solution for it to be fixed permanently.

For example, if you completely tear an anterior cruciate ligament (ACL) in your knee, you need an orthopedic surgeon. Nothing else is going to help much. The two injuries that almost always need surgery are ACL tears and superior labral from anterior to posterior (SLAP) tears.

If you have other kinds of pain, the causes are usually from your soft tissues such as fascia, muscles and tendons. Multiple different treatments can help with this. Their effectiveness depends on how good the therapist is and if the specific method is helping the root cause of your problem.

Fascia and scar tissue—You feel like your muscles are "hard" even when not contracted, or you have areas that feel "stuck" when you move. The best methods for this are active release, biomedical dry needling and the fascial abrasion tool.

Muscles not functioning well—you feel weak in certain muscles for no particular reason or your movements are not normal because of muscle dysfunction. Alternatively, you feel pain when performing certain movements. Dry needling, especially with electro-stimulation and trigenics, are good for this problem.

Trigger points and referred pain—These are tender spots in your body that cause pain in that area and perhaps in other areas (referred pain). I have found that dry needling is excellent for this. Self-massage or trigger point tools works well too.

Inflexibility—All of the above causes can lead to a loss in flexibility. This is especially noticeable when one side of your body moves better than the other does. Once the root problem is addressed as above, the best way to maintain flexibility is old-fashioned stretching. The best stretching method and one that is commonly used at my gym is called fascial stretching. This is designed by Ann and Chris Fredericks who are probably the top people in the world when it comes to knowledge about stretching.

If you have a problem get the right solution from the right therapist at the right time and your pain should get better rather quickly.

8.4 Common stretches

Note: All stretches are demonstrated on the book's website. It is very hard to teach with just words and pictures. Go to www.happybodybook.com to see how they are done.

These are the areas commonly "tight" in people because of inactivity or common posture problems. Many ideas about posture originate from the late Dr. Vladimir Janda's work. His ideas have stood the test of time as they originated in the 1970s–1980s. They are well recognized today but were truly ahead of their time when they first came out.

Stretching is a pretty broad subject, and there are hundreds of stretches to choose from, along with many different ways of performing them (From slow to fast to bouncing or swinging, with or without contractions in between stretches etc), which all have their uses in different situations. This section includes the commonly tight areas that need stretching in many people. These are not the only stretches that can be employed for these tight parts but they are ones that we commonly use, and that get excellent long-term results for our clients.

In my experience, I have noticed that women are far more faithful to their stretches than men are. Men try to give many excuses about why they don't need to stretch or why they don't have time. Women simply do it, even though stretching is not the most exciting or fun part of exercise. My team and I appreciate this about our woman clients because stretching is actually very good for you.

Before you start stretching, I like to use this technique with a foam roller to get better results. This technique is designed to gently release the muscles and fascia (connective tissues) of the chest all the way to the shoulders and hands (they are all connected!).

- Lie longitudinally on a foam roller with your legs bent and arms S-t-r-e-t-c-h-e-d out. There should be noticeable but not painful tension in the arms.
- Place a light object on the thumb side of your hands as you open the hands up.
- Make sure you have a relaxing environment.
- Lie here for at least twenty minutes.
- OPTIONAL: Change the angle of your arms to stretch different parts of your body. Vary them from closer to your side to up in a "Y" shape.

I know twenty minutes may seem like a long time but it does take at least twenty minutes to teach your body's nervous system that this new position is correct. After all, you may spend many hours a day driving, slouched in front of a computer or slumped in a chair. Twenty minutes spent to reverse this process is not too much to ask. If you can do forty minutes that would be even better! After this extended time, your body actually starts to use protein from your food to lay down tissue in this new, better position.

The opposite also is true; sitting, standing or slouching in a bad position for more than twenty minutes also teaches your body that this position is "normal" and it will be more difficult to reverse.

For pre-exercise stretches, follow the guidelines in **(12.3.2)**. The stretches listed here are to be done on rest days or before sleep because when done correctly they are relaxing. I like to use a form of what is called contract-relax stretching. Combined with relaxing breathing described in section **(4.3)**.

The general instructions for all of these stretches are as follows:

Step 1: Lightly tense up the muscle to be stretched for about five seconds (only a light 5-10% contraction is needed).

Step 2: Relax the muscle and breathe OUT while relaxing and going deeper into the stretch.

Step 3: Breathe lightly while holding this new, longer position for fifteen seconds.

Step 4: Repeat step 1 to 3 WITHOUT totally releasing the stretch. With each cycle allowing you to gently go deeper and deeper into the stretch. Once you find no more benefits by performing another cycle, then you can stop.

Step 5: Hold a mild tension stretch for three minutes or more. If you have time, you can hold it for twenty minutes or even longer! (perhaps 80% of the farthest you went with step 1 to 3). This is to "re-train" your nervous system to recognize the new position as normal.

Spend more time on your tighter side, and on stretches at which you are not good.

Note: If you have access to a good dry needling, ART, and/or trigenics practitioner, doing those procedures before stretching can multiply and speed up your results **(8.2)**.

8.4.1 Upper body

Pectorals 1
Start: Lie in the position shown.

    Step 1: Lightly tense up your chest muscles for about five seconds.

    Step 2: Relax and breathe out as you reach your arm and hand away from your shoulder and turn your body away from the arm.

    Step 3: Hold this position for fifteen seconds.

    Step 4: Repeat one to three times turning slightly farther away each time. For this stretch, remember to use different angles for your arm that is being stretched, from directly out, to up at approximately forty-five degrees.

Pectorals 2
Start: Get into the position shown using an exercise ball or bench that is at shoulder height.

    Step 1: Lightly tense up your chest muscles by pressing your elbow into the ball for approximately five seconds.

    Step 2: Relax and breathe out as you drop your shoulder joint. You should feel a stretch deep under your chest muscles.

    Step 3: Hold this position for fifteen seconds.

    Step 4: Repeat one to three times dropping your shoulder deeper each time. For this stretch, remember to use different angles for your arm that is being stretched, from directly out, to up at about forty-five degrees as shown in the picture. You can do this by moving your elbow that is on the ball or adjusting your body position.

Upper trapezius and scalene

Start: Perform standing, one arm behind back.

Step 1: Lightly tense up your muscles on the side of the neck against your hand for approximately five seconds.

Step 2: Relax and breathe out as you reach your back arm further down and back away from your shoulder while moving your neck further sideways.

Step 3: Hold this position for fifteen seconds.

Step 4: Repeat one to three times turning and moving your back arm further back and down while moving your neck further to the other side each time.

Step 5: Repeat this stretch without the arm behind your back. Simply put it on your hip for emphasis on the scalene (side of neck). You can also change the angle of your head slightly to target different fibers of these muscles.

Levator scapula

Start: Perform standing as seen in the picture.

Step 1: Lightly tense up your muscles on the side/back of the neck against your hand

Step 2: Relax and breathe out as you look down and toward your opposite foot.

Step 3: Hold this position for fifteen seconds.

Step 4: Repeat one to three times stretching your neck further down and across each time. You can also slide you other hand further down your hip each time.

Latissimus dorsi

Start: Perform standing as seen in the picture with a vertical object for you to grab, usually a doorframe works well.

Step 1: Lightly tense up the muscles in your back by pulling your upper arm's elbow lightly toward your hips (without moving your arm) for approximately five seconds.

Step 2: Relax and breathe out as you move your hips away from the doorframe.

Step 3: Hold this position for fifteen seconds.

Step 4: Repeat one to three times. You can turn your torso toward the floor and toward the ceiling slightly to get a different angle of stretch. Spend more time in the angles in which you feel tighter.

Pronator Teres

Start: Your right elbow is bent, and the right palm is turned up. Using your other hand, grab the thumb side of your palm from below as seen in the picture.

Step 1: Lightly tense up the muscle we want to stretch (it's in your forearm, near your elbow) by trying to turn your right palm face down against the resistance of your left hand for about five seconds.

Step 2: Relax and breathe out as you use your left hand to turn your right hand more palm up than in the start position, while extending your right arm.

Step 3: Hold this position for fifteen seconds.

Step 4: Repeat one to three times. Long holds for several minutes or more are a good choice for this muscle.

8.4.2 Lower body

Quadratus lumborum/IT band

Start: Perform lying on your side as seen in the picture.

Step 1: Lightly tense up the muscles on the bottom (floor) side of your body for about five seconds.

Step 2: Relax and breathe out as you straighten your arms, moving your chest further from the ground. Also, try to slide your bottom leg further down, away from your head.

Step 3: Hold this position for fifteen seconds.

Step 4: Repeat one to three times. You can turn your hips toward the floor and toward the ceiling slightly to get a different angle of stretch. Spend more time in the angles in which you feel tighter.

Lower back

Start: Perform lying face up.

Step 1: Tuck your knees to your chest then lightly contract your lower back by pushing your knees against your hands for about five seconds.

Step 2: Relax and breathe out as you straighten your arms and extend them outward while dropping your knees to one side.

Step 3: Hold this position for fifteen seconds.

Step 4: Repeat one to three times but do it to the opposite side.

Piriformis

Start: Lie face up with one foot on a vertical surface such as a pillar or wall.

Step 1: Put your right ankle on the thigh of the left leg. Lightly tense up the muscle you want to stretch by lightly pressing the right knee into your right hand.

Step 2: Relax and breathe out as you straighten your right arm, pushing the right knee away from you.

Step 3: Hold this position for fifteen seconds.

Step 4: Repeat one to three times. You can shift your buttocks towards the vertical surface for a greater stretch.

Hamstrings

Start: Lie face up with your hands behind your right knee.

Step 1: Lightly tense up the muscle you want to stretch by lightly pressing the right knee away into your hands.

Step 2: Relax and breathe out as you bend your arms, pulling your right knee toward you, at the same time trying to straighten your right leg completely. Don't worry if you can't do this at first. Just try your best.

Step 3: Hold this position for fifteen seconds.

Step 4: Repeat one to three times. You can shift your leg slightly to the left and right to stretch different parts of the hamstring.

Hip flexors

Start: Standing with your left foot on a chair or other raised surface.

Step 1: Lightly tense up the muscle you want to stretch by lightly contracting your right thigh and hip as if you wanted to drag your right foot forward but do so without moving your right foot.

Step 2: Relax and breathe out as you lift your right arm with palms up, do this while extending your chest upward, and sucking in your belly button a little.

Step 3: Hold this position for fifteen seconds.

Step 4: Repeat one to three times. You can arch back a little more and raise your hand a little higher each time for a greater stretch.

Thigh

Start: Kneel on the floor with your right foot elevated against an exercise ball. Place a towel or soft mat under your knee if necessary.

Step 1: Lightly tense up the muscle you want to stretch by gently straightening your right leg against the ball.

Step 2: Relax and breathe out as you raise your arms overhead while pushing your hips slightly forward. You should also suck in your belly button slightly.

Step 3: Hold this position for fifteen seconds.

Step 4: Repeat one to three times. You can shift your hips further forward and raise your arms even higher for a greater stretch.

Calves

Start: Stand about one meter from a wall or stabilizing surface with one foot in front of the other.

Step 1: Bend your back (right side) leg and lightly tense up the muscle you want to stretch by lightly pressing the right foot toes into the ground.

Step 2: Relax and breathe out as you bend your right leg as much as you can while keeping your heel on the ground to get a stretch in your right calf.

Step 3: Hold this position for fifteen seconds.

Step 4: Repeat one to three times.

Note: For calves, you need to do some stretches with your right toes turned slightly inward and slightly outward for different fibers in the calves. You will also need to do some stretches with your knee leg straight; also, a different part of the calves will be stretched. Finally, for calves, you do need to put a bit more weight into the stretches because the tissue there is quite thick in most people.

8.5 Common exercises

These are the areas commonly weak in people because of inactivity or posture problems. Training them will help hold posture and relieve stress on joints and pain. Muscles are like the hinges that hold one of those restaurant doors that can swing both ways. If either side is tight or weak, the door is stuck permanently in a misaligned position. Stretches and treatments help the short muscles, exercise and treatment help the weak ones.

Note: If you do the exercises with great technique but still can't feel the muscles, a fast fix is trigenics and or dry needling into the nerves that innervate these muscles. Needling with eletro-stimulation can be even more effective than needling alone. Ask your therapist about this.

8.5.1 Upper body

Lower trapezius

Start: Face down on a bench or bed with your head on your left fist. Your right arm is bent and your right hand is in front of your head with the thumb pointing up. Your shoulder blades are tucked up and inward.

End: Raise your right elbow and forearm one to two inches up and hold it there for five seconds. Perform twelve to fifteen repetitions.

Progression: Straighten your arm and perform the same movement. You can add resistance with weights in your hand once you can do the straight-arm version easily.

What you should feel: A tight contraction in the middle of your back near the spine.

Mid-trapezius

Start: Face down on a bench or bed with your head on your left fist. Your right arm is bent and dropping down off the edge of the bench. Your shoulder blades are tucked up and inward.

End: Raise your right elbow until it is slightly higher than your shoulder; hold it there for five seconds. Perform twelve to fifteen repetitions.

Progression: You can straighten your right arm, and then progress to add weight in your hand.

What you should feel: A tight contraction in the middle of your back at chest level, near the spine.

Rhomboids

Start: Face down on a bench with weights in your hands.

End: Bring the weights up at about chest height and tuck your elbows inward toward your torso at the finish position. Hold it here for five seconds. Perform twelve to fifteen repetitions.

Progression: Increase the weights you use, and/or increase the time that you hold the contraction at the top

What you should feel: A tight contraction in the middle of your back near the spine at chest level slightly deeper than the contraction for mid-traps.

Serratus anterior

Start: Start in an incline pushup position with you shoulder blades together.

End: With arms remaining straight, raise yourself by pushing your shoulder blades out. Hold it here for five seconds and lower under control. Perform twelve to fifteen repetitions.

Progression: Move to a flat position on the floor instead of an incline position.

What you should feel: tiredness in the side of your rib cage just in front of your armpits.

Supinator

Start: Right elbow bent, right hand palm down.

End: Using your left hand going over the top and grabbing the pinky side of your right palm resist your right palm, which is going to attempt to rotate palm up. Allow enough resistance with your left hand to let the right palm turn upward and then return downward slowly approximately five seconds up, and five seconds down. Perform ten to twelve repetitions.

Progression: Increase the resistance of your left hand, and or perform more repetitions.

What you should feel: tiredness in outside of your forearm of your right hand.

Lower fibers of abdominals

Start: Lie face up. Keep your back flat against the floor with your legs straight (if possible) and feet about six inches above the floor.

End: Hold this position for thirty to sixty seconds depending on your fitness level.

Progression: Add shoes, then later, ankle weights to make this more challenging.

What you should feel: Tiredness in the lower part of your abdominal muscles.

Transverse abdominnus

Start: Start in the all-fours position with a full breath of air.

End: Without moving your lower back at all, breathe out as you suck in your belly button and hold the "in" position for ten seconds. Repeat six to eight times.

Progression: Do this standing once you can do it in the all fours position without any movement in your lower back.

What you should feel: A tiredness deep in the abdominal region.

8.5.2 Lower body

Gluteous maximus

Start: Begin in the all-fours position.

End: Raise your right leg off the ground using only your butt muscles. If you feel tension in your hamstrings or lower back, do not lift the leg any further. Hold the contraction at the top position that you can reach for ten seconds. Then lower under control and repeat for six to eight repetitions.

Progression: Do this lying face up with knees bent, and feet on the floor. Contract your buttocks to thrust your hips up and hold the top position for ten seconds.

What you should feel: Tired in your buttock muscles.

Side of hips

Start: Begin lying on your side with legs straight.

End: Raise your top leg up as high as you can, and hold the top position for five seconds. Lower under control and repeat twelve to fifteen times.

Progression: Add ankle weights.

What you should feel: Tired at the sides of your hips.

Note: To get complete training of this area, make sure you vary the angle of your leg and foot position (sometimes leg slightly forward, sometimes leg slightly back, sometimes toes point up, sometimes toes point down).

VMO (8.6.3)

Tibialis anterior

Start: Sit on a bench with a dumbbell between your feet.

End: Raise your toes toward your face; hold the top position for five seconds. Lower under control and repeat twelve to fifteen times.

Progression: Increase the weight of the dumbbell.

What you should feel: Tired at the fronts of your lower leg.

8.6 Common pain fixes

If you have a choice, a trip to a good treatment specialist who understands your problem (8.3) is going to be the best way to solve a painful joint or area. However, there are many things you can do to take control of your recovery. These fixes are the key solutions that I have given clients over the years to help them solve and manage chronic pain.

8.6.1 Shoulder pain

Shoulder pain is one of the most common problems I see during health consultations. Most of the time the client tells me, "Oh it's been diagnosed as … tendinitis, rotator cuff tears, impingement" and so on. The problem is that the symptoms of shoulder pain feel about the same no matter which part of the shoulder is problematic. It is very hard to tell what the cause of the problem is just by description of the symptoms. The cause of shoulder pain is multi-multi-multi factorial. The reason for this is that the shoulder has more than twenty attachments and moving parts that affect its function. Any one of these or a combination of them can affect shoulder function and cause pain.

While you will require a well-trained therapist to check all the moving parts, some parts, in my experience, more commonly cause problems. Taking care of these can greatly reduce your risks of shoulder pain and if done progressively even if you are injured, they should improve some of your symptoms. As usual, never push into sharp pain, or dull pain that does not go away in a few seconds.

Step 1: *Improve your posture.*

If you slouch or hunch, your shoulders (and everything else) are in a mechanically weaker state and a more injury prone position. Chest up, head up posture is more attractive, projects more confidence and increases happiness. You don't see depressed people walking like that, and physical actions can change emotional states.

Good posture also is good for joints and muscles because it "stacks" your joints naturally one on top of the other so that the muscles work less hard against gravity to hold you upright. This leads to fewer strains and joint pain, as well as fewer tension-based headaches and backaches. In the case of your shoulder, it allows your shoulder blades to move more freely, which is important for almost any movement you can do with your arms, especially those that require you to move your arms overhead. The foam roller exercise for twenty minutes **(8.4)** is a good place to start. Correct breathing also is important **(3.3)**. The stretches and activation exercises in **(8.4)** and **(8.5)** also contribute greatly to posture.

Correct your habits.

- Tall

  Make yourself as "tall" as possible. You know, like in your school days when you were made to check your height each year? Yup. Just like that, we all made ourselves as "tall" as possible. This cue opens up the chest, gets rid of slouching, rotates your upper arms externally (palm up), as opposed to internally when we drive, type or read. It also points our chest forward and gets our head up and straight. In addition, try to turn your hands so that the thumb side edges of your hand point forward, instead of the back of the hand in most people who have poor posture.

- Thin

  Make yourself "thin." Imagine you are buttoning tight pants. You suck your belly button in slightly to make your tummy smaller. This activates the deep muscles of the abdomen that keep your hip and spine aligned. It prevents lower back problems and helps keep your pelvis level so that all the muscles around your hips can work in the most efficient way.

- Double chin

  I would say that the majority of people have rounded upper backs and a forward head position. That means that when they enter a room, their head enters before their chest. No matter your gender or pectoral development, your chest should enter a room before your head. To help fix this, make yourself a "double chin." This will be HARD for those of you who have been having the forward head position for a long time but work at it.

Step 2: Train the muscles that pull your shoulder blades back and down.

Most of us, because of common activities such as computer use, driving, and poor breathing habits, will tend to have what is called "overactive" muscles near our necks, which put our shoulder blades into a weakened position. One of the best exercises for this is shown below. It is actually a more advanced version of the lower trap exercise shown in **(8.5)**.

Instructions:
- Start with your head on your forearm, and the weight by your side.
- Shrug your shoulder blade back and down.
- Raise the weight into a "Y" shape with your thumb up, not straight ahead, and not out like a "T." The "Y" is the most difficult angle to move in and it's the one that needs the most training.
- Lower the weight under control for four to five seconds.
- You should feel the exercise in the middle of your back. That is where the muscles you want to train are (the lower trapezius muscles). If you don't feel it, decrease the weight, and try again. There is no point doing this if you don't feel the muscle.

Step 3: Train the muscles that rotate the shoulder.

These muscles taken together are called the "external rotators" of the shoulder, and are commonly very weak in many people. Their injury prevention function is in decelerating your arm movements, and stabilizing your shoulder joint. Because of the many angles in which your shoulder can function, there are hundreds of variations of this exercise using different positions and training equipment. Here is a simple one that almost anyone can do.

Instructions:
- Rest your elbow on something just below shoulder height. This is important because you don't want to use strength to lift your arm.
- Keep your elbow at ninety degrees, and lower the weight as far as you can without your shoulder rounding. Lower in four to five seconds.
- Bring the weight up by rotating your upper arm. You should not feel tired in your shoulder muscles but rather in the small muscles behind your shoulder. In fact, you should feel the exercise very much near your armpit. These are the small muscles we are trying to train here.

Step 4: _Train your biceps._

Many people ask "Why the biceps?" when I tell them that this is an important exercise. The reason is that part of the bicep muscle called the "long head" actually ends up inside the shoulder joint and connects to the tissue inside of the joint. This makes it a very important stabilizing muscle for the shoulder. When I test people with shoulder issues, the long head of the bicep is a common problem that needs to be addressed. To train the long head of your biceps, you will need a place to recline. Either an inclined bench or a gym ball should be okay.

Instructions
- Start with the arms straight and the elbows BEHIND your body.

- Start to curl the weights using your biceps; do not move your elbows at all.
- Once the forearms pass parallel with the floor, you can move your elbows a little forward to finish the exercise.
- Lower under control, reversing the movement, in four to five seconds.
- There we have it; do each exercise for four sets, with a load that is challenging for ten to twelve repetitions to start off. Your shoulders will be glad you did!

8.6.2 Back pain

Have any of you been camping? You know when you pitch a tent the incredible thing is that the tent is very strong and a good tent can even survive the night on a windy mountain slope. The secret to the strength of a tent is the poles or wires that anchor it to the ground. Without these poles or wires, the tent is just a flappy, weak piece of fabric.

It's the same thing with your spine. In general, my 85-year-old grandmother's spine can support about the same amount of weight as a world champion weightlifter. However, why do some people get injured picking up a pencil, while others can lift hundreds of kilos off the floor safely? The secret is in the strength of the muscles around the spine. World-renowned back health researcher Stewart McGill gives these following norms for core strength and stability that result in long-term back health.

The next time you are doing your exercise program, try these tests. They are fairly easy to do and are pretty safe. Because it is an endurance, rather than a strength test, the requirements are the same for men and women.

If you have problems holding the right position, or passing the test, it's time to use these exercises as part of your training so you can get your back and core strong enough to support your spine well so you can have a pain-free, and properly functioning back:

- back extension test,
- side bridge test, and
- front bridge test.

Tight hip flexors and weak glutes and quadratus lumborum are also common causes of back discomfort. So do the stretches and exercises for these muscles in **(8.4)** and **(8.5)** to get them sorted out as well.

8.6.3 Knee pain tips

Popliteus karate chop
This is a muscle activation trick that "turns on" the popliteus muscle behind the knee. This is a commonly problematic muscle that can lead to various kinds of knee discomfort both in front and back of the knee. The karate chop trick can help you deal with this. It is rather hard to describe in pictures so check out the video on our website www. happybodybook.com

VMO
Another commonly weak area of muscle surrounding the knees that we have found in most clients is the vastus medialis. Especially the oblique fibers of that muscle (VMO). This is the "teardrop" muscle that is on the inside of your knee. It stabilizes the joint and helps protect from injury. Yes ... in most people it doesn't look like a teardrop. That is because it is underdeveloped in almost everyone, and is hardly visible. This is because most sedentary people seldom get into a deep squatting position during training or daily activity where the VMO is turned on the most.

Don't worry; going all the way down in a squat exercise is safe. So is letting your knees pass your toes. Ask anybody who thinks it's dangerous to find a medical study dated after 1985 saying that it is dangerous. (Hint: such studies don't exist). In fact, studies on athletes who incorporate deep squats into their training program routinely show the best improvements in knee injury rates, as well as running and jumping ability.

The VMO is turned on the top and the bottom ranges of knee movement, so we need to load the top range of the movement as well as the bottom range. The two exercises we often use for the strengthening of the VMO for beginner clients are the incline step up and the split squat.

Below are descriptions of how to perform these two exercises correctly.

Incline step up
Start position:
- working foot on the board (in this case the left foot),
- other foot completely in front of the working foot,
- weight is on the balls of the working foot, and
- chest is upright.

Finish position:
- push your entire body-weight through the balls of your working foot to get to the finish position. Use ONLY the working foot, the non-working foot does not help you by "jumping."
- chest is up, look straight ahead; and
- the non-working foot stays in front.

If this is too easy, you can hold dumbbells in your hands to increase resistance. However, make sure you can perform it perfectly without wobbling, leaning forward or "jumping" off the non-working leg before increasing the resistance.

Split squats
After doing your incline step-ups or Peterson step-ups, you can do your split squats. The board under your front foot is optional and if you are strong enough and flexible enough, you don't need it.

Start position:
- chest up,
- long stride, and
- place feet with some "stagger" left and right. Imagine your feet are on a set of railroad tracks rather than on a single rail.

Bottom position
- Let your hips drop down AND forward.
- Let your knee go as far forward as possible.
- Make sure that your front leg "closes" completely. Imagine that there is something behind your front knee; your leg should squeeze it.
- Keep your chest up and look ahead.
- Your back leg should bend, and your back foot should point straight ahead rather than outward.
- To return to the start position move your head and shoulders BACK rather than lifting your buttocks and hips up.
- It is normal to feel a stretching in your back leg and hip.

Below is a picture of how your front foot should be positioned for the step up AND the split squat. It should be pointed about ten to fifteen degrees outward (see the foot on the board). This activates the quadriceps muscles better, and allows most people to get to a deeper and more comfortable bottom position.

Perform four sets of step-ups with twelve to fifteen repetitions per set. After that, perform four or five sets of split squats with ten to fifteen repetitions per set. Lower yourself in approximately four seconds and come up in two seconds.

Hamstrings

This exercise is called the hamstring curl. It uses a machine that is found in most decent gyms or fitness centers. Having strong hamstrings will help you keep your knees healthy. The reason is that hamstrings help your body absorb force when you run, jump, stop or turn. How? The hamstring muscles "wrap" around the knee joint keeping it more stable. In fact, part of your hamstrings even insert into your meniscus to help stabilize it (some fibers of the semi-membranosus insert into the medial meniscus). In addition, most physical therapists would see meniscus tears as a common knee injury. Long story short—strong hamstrings are a requirement for strong knees.

Start position:
- start with the roller or ankle pad of the machine under your Achilles tendon (just below your calves), and
- point your toes downward (like a ballerina).

You can vary your foot position to change the emphasis on different parts of your hamstrings. You can point them inward (as in the picture), straight or outward (like a penguin). I suggest most people start with the toes pointing inward as this is the weakest position for many clients and athletes. You can vary your foot position after a few weeks of doing them with toes inward.

Finish position
- bring your heels all the way up until you "kick" yourself in the buttock, and
- then lower the weight under control (approximately four to five seconds) to the starting position.

Note: Your calves may feel like cramping the first few times you do this. You will be tempted to point your toes up (toward your face). Don't do this. Instead, reduce the amount of resistance. When your calves feel like cramping, it is an indicator that you are too weak in the hamstrings, and your calves are trying to "help" but end up cramping instead.

Another thing you can do to improve you hamstring function is to stretch your hip flexors. Some of your hip flexors attach to your knee, so hip flexors that are of correct length will improve knee stability. This stretch is shown in **(8.4)**.

8.6.4 Upper back and neck aches

Here are the main areas that I have found that contribute most to neck and upper back discomfort. First, get your posture right **(8.6.1)**. Any time your head is "forward" of the rest of your body it imposes a much greater load on your neck and upper back. It is estimated that each inch that your head is forward of where it should be (it should be directly above your shoulders, imagine walking into a room, your chest should enter first, not your head), it can add about ten pounds (4.5kg) to the load on your upper back and neck muscles. Do this for an entire day and it is understandable why these muscles will give up under the strain.

The next problem area usually is the levator scapula muscle and the upper trapezius. The stretches for these muscles **(8.4.1)** should help you here. Also, the routine in **(8.6.5)** will help you as well.

Finally, you will want to work on the trigger points at your suboccipital, SCM and scalene muscles don't worry about the names, in the video we will show you how to massage these muscles effectively. They can be very tender and are common causes of back and neck pain and headaches.

8.6.5 Five minute coffee break routine

Here is what I would do at the office during a break to help relieve tension on commonly tight or overworked parts of your body. It will help to your body in balance despite the commonly poor positions of daily life.

- **For neck self-massage stretches and trigger points see— (8.6.4).**

- **Trigenincs upper trapezius release—see video.**
- **Chest expansion with external rotation.**

Start: Standing, bent forward at the waist with light stretch in your hamstrings.

End: "uncoil" your body, and stand up with your chest up, arms up in a "Y" shape, and palms rotated upward, making yourself as "tall" as possible. Repeat ten times slowly.

Chapter 9

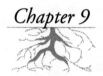

Nutrition

J amie is one of our clients who had tried many methods of weight loss including "detox in a box" plans, crash diets, and slimming pills. The problem was that the "quick fix" promises of many products do not follow the rules of how our bodies work, and as such, cannot give a long-term solution to healthy fat loss. After changing her nutrition to one that met the needs of her activity level, genetic history and foods she was tolerant of, she lost 16kg of fat in four months, and has kept it off for five months since then. She is so inspired to eat healthy food that she now runs a "food blog," which I direct new clients to for healthy recipes!

Key Point: There is no quick fix to nutrition problems but when you get it right, it works and you keep the benefits long-term.

This chapter will cover the basics of nutrition. It will help a person customize their nutrition for their body type, activity level and genetics.

This customization will help readers avoid the confusion over the large number of diet books and programs out there, which sometimes seem to give contradictory information.

Finally, a list of supplements that are helpful to replace missing nutrients from our food supply will be given. This will also help readers see through the misinformation of the unregulated supplement industry. This chapter will be slightly longer than most of the others, because if you get your fundamental nutrition principles right, many other problems start to resolve themselves.

9.1 Food is information

Before we begin, it is important to know something that is commonly misunderstood. Calories are not created equal. Food is not just a bunch of calories; it is also information telling your body what to do.

For example, this is a common daily food intake log from some of the nutrition consultations that I do for clients when they first visit our gym. There may be slight differences from country to country but the food choices will be similar.

- breakfast—bread with jam or other processed toppings, cereal, fruit juice, coffee;
- morning snack—biscuits from the office pantry or processed snacks from the store downstairs;
- lunch: rice, potato or pasta-based meal;
- afternoon snack—more pantry food like instant noodles; and
- late dinner is the same as lunch.

When I ask the person why he or she eats this way, *"Well, it's what everyone does"* is the main reason. That is the way an average person eats. True. However, remember … *average is not the same as normal.* This is not the way you should be eating normally for maximal health.

"But I have counted the calories, and it's within my recommended daily intake."

Calorie counting is not the most important thing, especially if you do not have the correct food type first. That is because food is not just calories. It is not even just nutrient content like grams of protein, fat or carbohydrates. In fact, food is information to tell your body what to do.

Problem 1: The bread, jam and cereals are high in refined carbohydrates, which tell your brain to relax and fall asleep.

Breakfasts like this are part of the reason many people have poor energy in the morning, and can't be productive at work. The best breakfast choice for most people is one I learned from Coach Poliquin; it is a piece of meat with a few nuts. At least have some food with protein like Greek yoghurt or eggs. Nuts and protein improve your concentration and memory **(6.2)**.

Problem 2: The biscuits and processed foods at snack time are usually full of refined carbohydrates (we just talked about those in problem 1) and refined vegetable oils and trans-fats.

Those oils signal your cell walls to become more resistant to nutrients entering the cell. This not only "starves" the cell but makes your blood sugar higher because, if the nutrients can't go into the cells, they stay in the blood. Eventually, these nutrients end up being stored in fat cells, which are always ready to accept them **(9.2.2)**.

A much better snack choice is some nuts (healthy fats) and perhaps some veggie sticks (a lot of fiber, which does not raise blood sugar). At lunch, besides the high refined carbohydrate content of white rice and pasta, the food quality often is compromised by unwashed vegetables and bad oils used in meat preparation. We have covered bad oils and refined carbohydrates but the unwashed vegetables in many food stalls still contain toxins. These toxins signal your body to slow its metabolism and store fat.

So, ideally, bring your own food to work. At least get some of those pre-bagged veggies from the supermarket and make sure you wash them yourself.

Problem 3: The late dinner signals your body to go into "digestion mode."

That is fine for most of the day, except that your liver is involved heavily in digestion and is not able to perform it's night time functions of detoxification and activating of hormones that repair your body and burn fat. This is why I suggest going to sleep slightly hungry.

As you can see, food tells your body what to do and that means food plays a huge part in determining what your body becomes. Quoting one of my mentors in nutrition and functional medicine, Dr. Bob Rakowski:

"The new science of nutrigenomics has proven that food is not just calories and micronutrients, it is information that drives genetic expression. All proteins—structural and enzymes are created by what we put into our body."

That is why one-thousand calories of meat, nuts and veggies is very different from one-thousand calories of French fries! Make good nutrition choices that are outlined in the following sections, and give your body the information and instructions to do the right things.

In the following segments, we will be discussing the basics about fat, protein and carbohydrates, all important to making good choices.

9.2 Fat

With a more recent and more complete understanding of how our bodies use and need fat for optimal function, fat has lost some of its "bad guy" image that was prevalent in the past, where it was blamed for everything from weight gain, to heart disease.

The wrong kinds of fat are still harmful but these fats are those that have been unnaturally processed or those eaten in the wrong amounts or in combination with refined carbohydrates.

9.2.1 Types of fat

There are many types of fat but in general, you can classify them into two categories according to their chemical structures. Within each category, there are many types coming from different kinds of food.

Saturated fats

The first category is saturated fats. These fats have been the most criticized as causes of disease. However, they do NOT cause problems by themselves. It is when they are not balanced with other kinds of fats like omega-3 and omega-9 unsaturated fats and when they are eaten in a diet full of refined carbohydrates and sugar, they cause a problem.

In fact, saturated fats are necessary for good health and from caveman times, have been an essential part of the diet for every healthy society. The long list of benefits below should be reason enough to keep unprocessed, saturated fats in your diet.

Saturated fats have awesome positive effects:

- increased good types of HDL **(5.5)**;
- decreased lipoprotein (another risk factor for heart disease);
- increased brain development in children;
- increased strength from better nerve connections;
- lowered blood sugar (when used with a low carbohydrate diet);
- increased bone strength because saturated fat is required for calcium use;
- increased nutrient absorption because many nutrients are fat soluble;
- improved liver health, which lowers abdominal fat levels;
- improved lung health because saturated fat is needed for the lining of the lungs;
- improved immune system function as some saturated fats have anti-viral properties (they actually destroy the cell walls of viruses, yay!); and

- improved digestive tract function because natural saturated fats encourage good gut bacteria.

Unsaturated fats

Now we move on to the second category, unsaturated fats.

The most important kinds of unsaturated fats are those that your body in unable to make on its own. You have to eat them to get them. The two kinds of unsaturated fats that you need are omega-3 and omega-6.

What makes them so important is that they not only provide energy but they also provide the following benefits. These mostly relate to omega-3 intake because most people have excess omega-6 in their processed and non-organic foods:

- production of Eicosanolids, which perform signaling duties in your body regulating things like immune system, heart rate, blood pressure and inflammation response;
- increasing insulin sensitivity and lower blood sugar;
- improving communication between cells;
- improves mood and brain function

increases quality of arteries;

- turn on fat burning genes and enzymes; and
- turn off fat storage genes.

In fact, they have a positive benefit on every disease known to humankind—a list too long for any book!

So, where do we get these healthy fats? Here is a list of foods that have excellent sources of saturated fats:

- cream,
- butter,

- coconut oil,
- grass fed/free range meats, and
- eggs with yolk.

Unsaturated fat sources
Omega-3 (Get them from animal sources as they are more readily usable by the body.)

- fatty fish (e.g., salmon, mackerel, sardines);
- krill; and
- grass fed/free range meats.

Omega-9

- nuts of all kinds and seeds;
- olive oil; and
- sunflower oil.

Omega-6 (Limit these, as they are very commonly found, and excessive omega-6s lead to increased inflammation and disease risks)

- all vegetable oils,
- nuts, and
- farm raised animal meats (non-free range).

CHARTS: From L3 guide

9.2.2 The problem with trans-fats …
Trans-fat is the worst kind of fat. Trans-fats lower good HDL types, increase total cholesterol, bad forms of LDL cholesterol, triglycerides, VLDL, blood clots, risk of all heart conditions, blood pressure, obesity, blood sugar levels, insulin resistance and brain diseases and shrinkage!

Why? It's an unnatural fat with the same content but different "arrangement" than natural fat sources. Your body has NO CLUE what to do with this trash and just stores it and uses it to build cell walls and other structures. It also is very stable so it stays stored for a long time. So, the best idea is never to take it in.

Sources—Baked goods, chips, crackers, deep fried foods, fries, and anything that says margarine or hydrogenated oil.

9.3 Carbohydrates

Carbohydrates are possibly the most "confusing" nutrient to get right. There are bodybuilders and lean athletes who already swear by the benefits of carbohydrates (they are right!) and there are people with pre-diabetes, heart conditions or metabolic syndrome who are (correctly) given very low carbohydrate diets by excellent doctors and well informed personal trainers.

The previous paragraph was not a contradiction. Both groups of people are probably eating the right carbohydrate amounts for their goals and current health status. As you might have guessed, it is the individual person's current situation that determines the right carbohydrate intake for him or her.

To start with, our physiological requirement for carbohydrates is ZERO. That's correct; we don't actually "need" them at all to stay alive. If I had a room of one-thousand people and I divided them into three groups, with one group given zero fats, one group given zero protein, and one group given zero carbohydrates, it would be painfully obvious within a few weeks that the health of the zero carbohydrate (but healthy amounts of other nutrients) group would be doing fine.

On the other hand, the health of the other two groups would deteriorate rapidly. If I checked on them after a year, I suspect most of the zero protein and zero fat group would be very sick, or dead, while the zero carbohydrate group would still be doing okay! After all, as Weston Price, the famous researcher of indigenous groups of people noted even in the early 1900s, cultures could do very well with great energy, virility and health on very low carbohydrate diets.

As you will see, carbohydrates still have their place, and this section will explain how to add them to your diet. Before getting into how to choose the right amount of carbohydrates for your needs, here are the key things to know about carbohydrates.

9.3.1 Glycemic index and load

A common trend among people giving nutrition advice is that we should eat low glycemic index carbohydrates most of the time. This is only partially correct. For example, carrots and watermelon have a high GI (in the 80–90+ range), so in theory they are not good for you. They are close in GI rating to pure sugar, which is rated at 100. On the other hand, spaghetti has a GI of about 50.

Therefore, in theory, spaghetti is a much better choice of carbohydrate than carrots or watermelon. However, upon close inspection, when glycemic LOAD is considered, this is not the case.

Glycemic load is found by multiplying the glycemic index by the amount of carbohydrates in a typical portion size of that food.

- A portion of carrots or watermelon has between 5–8g of carbohydrates so its glycemic load is (assuming 7g per portion, and a GI of 90) 7*90/100=6.3, which is low.
- Alternatively, a portion of spaghetti has about 50g of carbohydrates. With a GI of 50, the glycemic load is 50*50/100 = 25 which is high.

From your own experience, you will probably note that this is true. Many overweight people love spaghetti and other pasta but how many overweight people have carrots or melons as their favorite food? From the more accurate GL comparison, carrots are a better choice for health as you would need to eat a bucket of carrots to equal a plate of pasta.

CHARTS: GL GI for carbs

9.3.2 Carbohydrate continuum

In practice, it is hard to know the glycemic index or glycemic load of every food. While some online apps can help, there are times where you find a food about which you are not sure. Below is a simple way to make a good guess about whether you should or should not be eating a particular carbohydrate.

Not all carbohydrates are created equal. They have different effects on our blood sugar and fat storage mechanisms. Here is the order in which we teach clients to choose carbohydrates. They are arranged in general, from low to high glycemic load and in terms of the effects they have on fat storage and overall health.

Carbohydrate levels
1. green vegetables of all kinds;
2. non-green vegetables and berries;
3. low fructose and low GI/GL fruits (apricots, apples, pears, citrus fruits, avocados, peach, tomatoes);
4. higher fructose/GI/GL fruits (papaya, banana, cherries, grapes, melons, mangoes, pineapples);
5. unprocessed starches (yam, sweet potatoes, brown rice, quinoa, chick peas, beans, sprouted grain bread);
6. "white" starches—white potatoes, rice and all flours; and
7. nonsense processed foods (everything else).

Who should eat what?

- If you are naturally lean and can handle starches well, stay at numbers one to five with an occasional six if you have no grain-related allergies.

If you are a natural fat boy (oops, that includes me ...) stay within numbers one to three for best results.

- If you are overly fat (can't see your abs at all)—more than 20% for women and 15-18% for men, then stay within one and two.
- Adjust according to your activity level. The more active you are, the more you can eat some of five and six, especially after a hard training session.
- Number seven is a bad idea in general!

9.3.3 Glycation

Glycation is a big contributor to aging, and is caused by carbohydrates. In particular, refined carbohydrates, and the most guilty one of all being high fructose corn syrup (HFCS). HFCS is touted by many food companies as similar to sugar and often is used as a substitute for sugar as it is cheaper to produce. HFCS is handled much more slowly in your body than regular sugar and thus ends up hanging around like the drunk person who just won't leave the party.

The problem with this is that HFCS has a tendency to connect and get stuck to the protein structures in your body to form what are known as "advanced glycation end products" (AGES—quite aptly named I would say...), which are proteins that have been damaged by sugars.

Just imagine a healthy piece of meat, which represents the many protein-based parts of your body. What does a good piece of meat feel like when it is raw? It feels slippery and smooth. That is what your protein structures should feel like.

However, having damaged glycated proteins in your body is like baking your meat in honey and teriyaki sauce, which represent excess fructose. The meat becomes sticky and no longer feels like meat.

This makes the proteins unable to perform their functions properly. If it's in your eyes, you get cataracts more easily, if it's in your brain, you get Alzheimer's more easily, if it's in your cardiovascular system, you get heart disease and diabetes more easily and so on.

Common sources of HFCS:

- sodas and soft drinks,
- candy,
- most cereal,
- syrups,
- bread,
- condiments (e.g. BBQ sauce and ketchup),
- pre-made desserts, and
- yoghurt—used to preserve the fruit in yoghurt, negating its beneficial effects on digestion.

Other names used to "hide" HFCS—some foods may try to hide HFCS under other names. Don't be fooled:

- inulin,
- glucose-fructose syrup,
- iso-glucose,
- chicory, and
- fruit fructose.

Overall, AGES are just another reason that you really want to stay away from HFCF and refined carbohydrates.

8.4 Protein

Protein is critical to your body. It builds enzymes, hormones, immune system and acts as a transporter for nutrients and oxygen, it also repairs tissue and can be used for energy.

Protein is made up of different kinds of amino acids, much as words are made up of alphabets. There are three kinds of amino acids, essential, non-essential and conditionally essential. Essential amino acids cannot be produced from other amino acids. Non-essential amino acids can be produced from other amino acids and conditionally essential amino acids can be made under special conditions.

As with essential fats, you cannot produce protein from fats or carbohydrates, so you do need to eat protein. In addition, you are not able to store amino acids so you need to eat protein consistently.

Sources of protein that contain all of the essential amino acids are called "complete" protein sources. These are usually animal-based proteins from meat and dairy products. The only known plant that I recommend with a complete protein profile is the South American seed called quinoa.

There are several methods that try to measure the absorbability of proteins. However, each of these methods have their pros and cons that lead them to be less than totally accurate. In the end, eating a wide variety of mostly animal-based proteins is your best bet for a wide spectrum of amino acids and maximum benefits for your health.

Protein is great for fat burning because it is filling and it is "expensive" to burn, requiring about 30% of its own energy to digest itself, leading to greater metabolism and energy expenditure.

There is a huge variance in the protein needs of a person, including things such as:

- level of body fat,
- gender,
- amount of lean muscle,
- activity level,
- pregnancy,
- age,
- illness, and
- stress.

For the general population, simply having a planned sized portion of seafood or meat three times per day is a good start. This needs to be adjusted according to the factors given above **(9.6.4)**.

9.5 Water

Water intake is one of those things … if you have to ask, you probably aren't drinking enough of it - and drinks other than water don't count! The benefits of water are abundantly clear and have direct impact on how well the rest of your lifestyle changes happen. I'm not just talking about surviving and avoiding dehydration; I'm talking about giving your body enough to thrive.

Well hydrated joints hurt less, a well hydrated digestive tract doesn't get constipated, well hydrated muscles contract harder, well hydrated fat cells shrink faster, and well hydrated brain cells work better and there is good evidence that a well hydrated body has lower risk for almost all diseases from diabetes to heart conditions to cancer.

Drinking the correct amount of water each day also fills your stomach, which sends an "I'm full" signal to your brain, reducing cravings for food.

Note: be especially aware of dehydration as you age, because the kidneys and water regulating hormones decline with age. In fact, even your thirst sensation decreases with age and you run a higher risk of dehydration. If you are going to exercise, a good tip is to make sure that you weigh more at the END of your training session than at the start. That's a good sign that you have not lost too much water.

Amount

The minimum amount of water you aim to take in should be somewhere in the region of 35-40g/kg of weight. That means a 50kg (110 pounds) woman should be drinking at least 1.8 liters (60 ounces) of water per day. But this is a bare minimum. Add more if you are … sick, live in a cold country, live in a hot country, exercise a lot or carry low body fat. A woman that size in a tropical country like mine should be taking in about 3 liters of good quality water each day for maximum benefits.

Water quality

Where you live in the world, as well as the age and reliability of your water distribution system makes a big difference in the quality of the water you are drinking. In general, water near agricultural regions (pesticides and fertilizer run-off) and industrial areas (heavy metal and plastics) are worse. Be aware of nearby activities as they also affect water quality, for example, areas near airports or air force bases have a higher possibility of benzene (i.e., jet fuel) in the ground water and agricultural areas tend to have some pesticide runoff.

Because of this inconsistency, I recommend getting a good water filter that does a few things:

- disinfects with UV light (kills stuff like E. coli and cryptosporidium bacteria);
- filters to get rid of heavy metals (like mercury, lead and cadmium);
- ionizes and alkalizes the water to concentrate the useful minerals (concentrates all the good minerals in the output water); and
- improves your body's antioxidant capacity and alkalinity.

From experience, two good brands that my colleagues and I have used with success are Akai (Japan), and KYK (Korea).

9.6 Putting your nutrition plan together

As Albert Einstein correctly said, "Insanity is doing the same thing over and over again and expecting different results." A big part of the reason many people have health issues that are addressed in this book, is because of poor diet. If health is going to change, a change in food is needed. This can be a bit daunting because of two main things.

One: Habits

The way we eat could have been the way we have "done things" since we were a kid. Comfort foods, family traditions, and often even the guilt of turning down gifts of food and snacks.

Two: Misinformation/Confusion

Eating fat is bad; you need to eat a lot of dairy products to get calcium, don't eat egg yolks, and whole grains are excellent foods.

In my experience, getting over these two factors are especially true when helping female clients. I believe that this is because women are better listeners than men! This is a wonderful character trait. However, it can be taken advantage of by unethical or uninformed companies and advertising to try to sell women methods and products that are often more hype than results (at best), or in many cases, damaging to their health.

Here are the steps my team and I use to change a person's nutrition. If you are more than 15% fat for men, and 20% for women, or more than 5kg (eleven pounds) from your desired weight, I suggest a fourteen-day "boot camp" program **(9.6.2)** to get your body kick-started into a healthy fat loss mode.

9.6.1 Can I eat this food? Just ask these two questions.

Any time I have a client ask me, "Can I eat this food," I ask them to ask themselves two basic questions.

Question 1: "Did a caveman have access to this food, in this form?"

If a caveman could get it, it's probably good for you, if he did not, it's probably bad for you. If a caveman could get his hands on it, it is most likely real food, and unprocessed. That means your body is able to use it and is unlikely to store it as fat.

For example, a caveman could get poultry (he could hunt and trap birds) but he did not have access to chicken nuggets. He had access to root vegetables like sweet potatoes but he did not have sweet potato pies!

Question 2: "Does this food have an advertisement?"

Simply put, every step of food processing adds profit but usually takes away nutritional value from the food. The more processed the food is, the more money the food company makes, and the more they have for advertising. Ad space is brutally expensive, so once you see an ad on television, in a magazine or on the side of a bus, you know that there is a huge profit margin on that food. This is good for stockholders of the big food companies but probably bad for you.

For example … do you see advertising for carrot juice? Probably yes. How about raw carrots? You almost never see those—because carrots are good for you but watered down, reduced fiber, chemically enhanced, sugar boosted, high profit fruit juices are not.

9.6.2 STEP 0: Start with two weeks of nutrition "boot-camp"

Boot-camp guidelines:

- take a "before" photo **(1.3)**;
- an unlimited amounts of caveman meats can be eaten, no need to stuff yourself but do feel satisfied. This includes seafood and fish and eggs (once per week);
- an unlimited amount of green vegetables and one to two servings of berries per day;
- one handful of any kind of nuts for women and two handfuls for men each day;
- generous amounts from other sources of healthy fats (four to six tablespoons)—see table;
- water intake at least the amount calculated as per section above;
- coffee—one to two cups per day, with cream not milk, add cinnamon if desired, organic if possible.

- absolutely no: grains, starchy carbohydrates, diary, alcohol; and
- after two weeks, have a refeed meal and then follow the steps outlined below.

The reason for the two-week boot camp is to make your body "fat adapted." This means that you need to start learning to use fat as a good source of fuel. In the past, most people, because of a diet full of refined carbohydrates, tend to use carbohydrates as their primary source of fuel. In such a situation, your body will not use its fat stores as fuel, so it will be hard to burn off that fat on your tummy or thighs. What we need to do is to turn on the entire "fat burning" machinery in your body—digestive enzymes, hormones and the entire energy production system in your cells.

This takes some time. It would be similar to a factory, which makes, for example Toyota cars, being asked to make iPods instead because they are more profitable. The factory cannot simply switch from cars to consumer electronics in a day. The workers need to be retrained, the machines need to be retooled and the supply processes need to be adjusted. This is what is happening in your body when you start to use fats as a good source of fuel instead of carbohydrates.

If you are just a few kilos, or a few percent body fat from your idea fat level, you may not need the boot camp period although it is not harmful to try it out. You can just go straight into the healthy steps listed below.

9.6.3 Step 1: Adjust food types

You will still need to eat unprocessed foods. Follow the caveman food choices and principles as outlined above. With the following difference, if you have a hard training session, then add some "Level 5" carbohydrates **(9.3.2)** only during your post-training window, within thirty minutes of the end of your training. For a woman or a man under 80kg, one serving (one bowl of rice, or one large potato) should be enough. Larger males can have up to two servings. Carbohydrates eaten post-training tend to have great benefits for refilling muscle energy, and will usually not harm fat burning if you are not overweight.

As with all things, it's best to check. So, use one of the fat measurement methods (2.3) to see if your current post-training carbohydrate intake is working well. If it is, you will see weekly reductions in body-fat and usually waist measurements as well.

Commonly allergenic foods

Also, make sure that you remove commonly allergenic foods, which can derail your healthy lifestyle plans even if you have the best intentions and the above factors in place.

While the best way to find out which foods are allergenic for you is a blood test (Chapter 10), you can get a good head start by removing the commonly disruptive foods:

- wheat,
- soy,
- diary,
- shellfish,
- eggs, and
- peanuts.

Finally, you can add supplements, which aid health and fat burning (9.8).

Do step one for a few weeks and measure to see how your results are. If they are good, keep going to step two. Make sure to do step one until you are at least 90% compliant (i.e. nine out of ten meals are good before moving on).

9.6.4 Step 2: Adjust food quantity

Protein goal.
Next, you need consistently to hit your protein goals using healthy meats and fish of all kinds. If you are training, try to hit at least 1-1.2g per pound of weight for men, and 0.9-1g per pound for women. Split this up so that you get some protein in every meal.

Add in carbohydrates or fats depending on current status.
Start with 50g of carbohydrates per day post-training as in Step 1. If you are getting leaner with 50g per day, slowly add carbohydrates back into your diet in steps of 10g per day, per week (e.g., this week 50g per day, next week 60g, and 70g the week after that), increasing only if you continue to get leaner. If not, go back to the previous week's amount. Use high quality, natural, unprocessed carbohydrates.

Two things to note, first, you can eat these additional carbohydrates any time other than post-training. I suggest late in the day as they help relaxation and sleep. Second, you don't need to count carbs from green veggies as part of your quota since they are mostly fiber, which doesn't affect blood sugar much.

Amounts still matter.
I had a client in the past who had trouble losing weight despite a healthy "caveman" diet and a challenging gym workout. When I asked her about food, she told me about all the healthy food she was eating (e.g., veggies, lean meat, seafood, omega-3 oils). Then I asked her about nuts. "Oh I eat a big bag of those while watching television with my husband at night."

That was the problem.

Yes, nuts are healthy but no, you can't eat half a kilo of them per day and expect to drop body fat effectively. It is simply too much food.

On the other hand, there isn't much point adjusting food quantity if you don't change food types as well. For example, eating 1500 calories of French fries (you will still be fat!) is completely different from eating 1500 calories from meat, nuts, fruits and veggies (you will get leaner).

Remember from **(9.1)** that food is not just calories; it also is nutrients and information. Nutrients tell our bodies to "feel full." It is possible to be overfed, yet malnourished because our bodies don't notice calories as much as they notice nutrient levels. If you ate 1500 calories of veggies and protein, you will be far more full than if you ate 1500 calories of chips, cakes or cookies. Why? Refined flour products (and other processed foods) have far fewer nutrients, and are full of more calorie dense bad fats and carbohydrates, so your body doesn't signal that it is full because it's not well nourished. Nutritious food, signals "full" far sooner.

Keep bad stuff away
Here are some tips to help you keep from excess eating of unhealthy foods. These are research-based tips and I learned them from the excellent, researched-based self-development book *59 Seconds*.

- Keep your food in opaque containers—research shows that food kept in opaque containers was less likely to be eaten than food kept in the open, or in clear containers.
- Keep your food further away—food kept within arm's reach was eaten more!
- Smaller spoons—Subjects who were given a smaller spoon ended up eating less
- Smaller bowls—We tend to finish what's on our plates or in our bowls, in studies where bowls were secretly refilled, subjects who had "secret refills" seemed to get less full and simply kept eating.
- Mirror in kitchen—A mirror in the kitchen or in a place where you dine increases body awareness and subjects who were in a place with a mirror they could see themselves in while deciding what, and how much to eat, tended to eat roughly 32% less.

Note: Do Step 2 until you are 90% compliant with both Step 1 and 2. If you don't get these two things consistently right, moving to Step 3 doesn't make a lot of difference.

9.6.5 Step 3: Adjust food timings

Once your food choices and food amounts are in order, you can work on food timings.

In general: Eat meat and nuts and healthy fats for breakfast.

Choose your carbohydrate types **(9.3.2)** and amounts **(9.6.4, 9.6.5)** then start adding them in at different times in the following sequence. Once again, do this for two weeks and then re-measure yourself, or take a photo again **(1.3)**.

- Start by adding in almost all of your carbohydrates after exercise.
- If you keep getting leaner add the additional carbs, determined in **(9.6.4)** by increasing 10g/week, at your evening meal.
- If you are getting leaner, keep increasing the total carbs **(9.6.4)** and split them between the evening and the pre-workout meals.
- If you are still getting leaner, you can even have some low GI/ GL carbs in the morning as well, usually in the form of fruit.
- Any time you find from your measurements or pictures, that you stop getting leaner, go back one step.
- Don't eat too much fat after training. Try to make post-exercise meals carbohydrates and protein (fish and rice for example, rather than pork belly and rice).

Go to bed slightly hungry. It's okay to eat at night but I prefer not to do "don't eat XYZ hours before sleep" rules because they don't make much sense. I may tell you to avoid food two hours before bed but if you sleep at 11pm and eat a buffet at 9pm, you will still not get many benefits.

What is actually happening is that if you sleep slightly hungry, during sleep your liver can focus on things that help you burn fat, like activating the right hormones, and detoxifying your body. If you eat a lot before bed, your liver will be overworked, as it also is involved with digestion.

9.6.6 Step 4: Maintenance

Now is the time to keep all the habits that you have built up. The important thing to fight fat gain in the long run, is to be aware without being obsessive. I suggest weighing yourself once per week, on the same scale, at the same time, on the same day.

Let's say you choose to measure every Monday morning before work. If this reading goes up more than 1 kg, it's time to decrease carbohydrate and/or caloric intake slightly for a few days and get yourself back on target. Re-measure the next week.

Remember, fat releases hormones and enzymes that keep fat in business, so the best time to fight fat gain is at the very first pound or kilo!

9.6.7 Troubleshooting

If you have followed the boot-camp program and done Steps 1 through 4, you should be well on your way to excellent results. If things are stuck, don't worry; here is the procedure to overcome stalled fat loss efforts.

Check your compliance.

Sometimes you might think you are complying with all the guidelines. However, the standard to meet is quite high—90% compliance. That means, out of ten meals that you eat, nine of them have to be following the guidelines of this chapter.

Check your food quantities.

Yes, you can eat a lot of healthy food but it is still possible to stay or get fat eating healthy food. After all, even if I eat completely organic and healthy food choices but I eat 10,000 calories per day, I will still be fat. Just to be sure, use a free online food tracking software like "myfitnesspal.com" to check your food intake. For fat burning, try to hit about eleven to twelve times your weight in pounds in calories (e.g., a two-hundred pound man would want to hit 2200 to 2400 calories per day).

Check your other health markers.

Do you as Dr. Rakowski says, "Eat right, sleep right, talk right, think right, drink right, move right, poop right." Is there anything in that list that is not going well? Get that sorted out either with your qualified coach or doctor.

Repeat until successful.

9.6.8 Meal preparation tips

If you want the best results, it will be best to prepare your food on your own. In this way, you are in total control of the ingredient content and quality of the things that you eat. Here are some tips.

- Shop twice per week for vegetables, and once or twice for meats.
- Buy only healthy items. Anything unhealthy will almost certainly be eaten. You will find these on the outside edges of supermarkets. Almost everything on the "inner" lanes is probably better for you.
- Prepare foods in big batches. Cooking and cleaning one pot of food is not much harder than cooking and cleaning one plate of food. Store some of the remainder in the freezer and heat it up when needed.

- Some sources of good, healthy recipes fit the nutrition recommendations in the book. There are also many websites with free recipes.
- Books:
  » *Nourishing Traditions*—Sally Fallon
  » *Gourmet Nutrition*—Dr. John Berardi and team
  » *The Paleo Diet Cookbook*—Dr. Loren Cordian
  » *Primal Blueprint Quick And Easy Meals*—Mark Sisson
- Websites:
  » everydaypaleo.com
  » nomnompaleo.com

9.7 Genetics

We all know that people come in all shapes and sizes. The differences can be very large. On one of my trips to attend a seminar, I met a guy who played professional American Football. He could bench press 140 on an incline bench for eight repetitions as a warm-up. His shoulders were almost as wide as the gym machine he was on, just about everything about him was big, even his fingers, nose and head. No matter how much I train, and even if I used illegal anabolic steroids, I am physically incapable of achieving that sort of size.

We have had a client who weights 85kg, has sub 7% body-fat (veins in thighs and calves and a nice six-pack of abs) is strong and has a very nice looking physique.

He eats only two meals per day—or sometimes one. He eats average quality food, he trains with average consistency and he sleeps only four to five hours per night. That sounds easy! Why can't we all do that? Simple … genetically, we are less gifted. He can—we cannot. Myself included.

He has an excellent metabolism, high levels of muscle building and fat burning hormones, strong detoxification ability and very good ability to tolerate carbohydrates of all kinds. The rest of us have to be more consistently good with our nutrition and lifestyle plans, detoxification plans and sleep habits even to get close to the physique that such a gifted individual has. It can be done but it just takes more love—love of being healthy, strong and fit.

World record sprinter Usain Bolt's meal before he broke the 100m world record at the 2008 Olympics was Chicken McNuggets. That is by no means ideal nutrition, but he broke (totally smashed) the world record. He can—we cannot.

Michael Phelps, the man with the most Olympic medals ever, eats a high processed carb, high starch, 12,000 calorie per day diet and wins multiple medals in Olympic swimming. (He also has long arms and flipper-like double jointed, big feet). He can—we cannot.

I hope all of this doesn't discourage you! As an encouragement, I too am a former fat boy who is by no means a genetically gifted athlete. However, being less gifted helps me to be more determined and diligent in searching for the best methods to help clients with more challenging nutrition and health.

9.8 Supplements

The benefits of supplements have been hotly debated; I hope I can provide some perspective on their usefulness along with recommendations for useful general health supplements. If a supplement is used specifically for a certain problem or condition, it is covered individually in that part of the book.

9.8.1 Do we actually need supplements?

The answer is, "It depends." In fact, although my gym does sell supplements, I really do wish we didn't need them because that would mean we live in a much healthier world. You probably don't need supplements:

- if you live in a clean place with minimal pollution;
- if you have a lifestyle where you get enough sleep;
- if you have a job that is not very stressful;

- if you have plenty of healthy and positive relationships with people;
- if you have access to, and almost always eat free-range, wild meats and plant foods grown in healthy soil; and
- if you have good genetics for detoxification.

If you have most or all of the above, you probably don't need many (if any!) supplements.

Unfortunately, this is not the case for much of the world's population, especially if you live in a big city or in a place where there is environmental damage from mass farming and industry. Since most of us don't live in such a "garden of Eden" kind of pristine environment, we will almost certainly have nutritional deficiencies. If we cover these deficiencies with supplementation we will get noticeable health benefits.

It also is important to remember that there is probably no "ideal" amount of each nutrient required for each person. Aside from the basic FDA daily requirement to prevent disease, there also is a "functional" difference in the amount of nutrients each person requires.

For example, a person who has lived in a place where magnesium rich foods are abundant (so he is used to having a lot), will probably need more for his individual needs than someone who's body is conditioned to a lower magnesium intake. If he also is doing a lot of exercise, sweating a lot because he is in a hot climate, and is under stress at work, these needs become even greater. This is where laboratory testing **(Chapter 10)** can really help a person determine what he needs more, or less of, thus getting a better outcome, and saving time and money in the long run.

9.8.2 Which brands are trustworthy?

The supplement industry largely is unregulated. This means a lot of low end companies try to make money before it is found out that their product doesn't work (or might even be harmful). As a consumer, this becomes a problem because it is not really possible to tell the difference between a high quality product versus a low quality one simply by looking at the label, the bottle, or even the capsule itself.

However, several companies hold themselves to higher standards and choose the suppliers of their ingredients properly. They also put research and thought into how they formulate their products and they sell their products mostly through licensed medical professionals. The price of these products would certainly be a little more. However, the quality, safety, potency and absorbability of their contents more than make up for the extra cost.

While I may not know every company of this kind that exists, here are some companies that I trust because I have had the pleasure of meeting with their education team, their product design team or the health care professionals who endorse their product. Each of these brands carry some similar products, and some items such as their omega-3 oils may even come from the same sources but they usually have several products that are special to their brand:

- *Poliquin*—endorsed by Olympic coach Charles Poliquin,
- *Designs for Health*—a good range of high quality formulas,
- *Pure Encapsulations*—has some of the highest rated ingredients and their own manufacturing facilities,
- *Metagenics*—high quality products with an excellent education team,
- *Wise Woman Herbals*—some of the best herb preparations I have used with clients, and
- *Life Extension Formulas*—excellent information on their website and in their free magazine. Their products can sometimes be found in higher end stores. Probably the best brand you can get "off the shelf" in a supplement store.

There are too many brands out there for anyone to know everything about that brand but if you can't get hold of the brands listed above there are a few ways to find out if a brand puts quality and effectiveness ahead of making a quick buck from an uninformed customer.

Here are three things to look out for.

Check their mineral supplements.

(Just Google their product name) and look for the way they add in minerals like magnesium and zinc. A cheap brand would add in a form like "oxide" (e.g., zinc oxide). A good brand would add in a mixture of "ate" forms (e.g. zinc orot-"ate" and magnesium glycin-"ate"). So, a magnesium supplement may have a mixture of magnesium glycinate, magnesium aspartate and magnesium citrate.

These "ates" mean than the mineral is connected to an amino acid transport mechanism, which leads to far greater absorption than the oxide form. Also, a brand that includes a mixture of different "ates," tends to absorb better because each "ate" form tends to go toward different kinds of tissue so no single tissue gets saturated. This also is good for the absorption of the mineral. After all, it's not about how much you eat; it's about how much you can absorb.

Check their vitamin E.

Another good indicator that a company cares that its supplements work rather than that they simply sell is the quality of their vitamin E. Vitamin E has many (eight) forms, and all of the forms are needed together for you to get the benefits related to vitamin E. Most cheap supplements simply add in synthetic "alpha-tocopherol" which is the simplest way to put something into a supplement and qualify to call that "vitamin E." An unsuspecting customer wouldn't know the difference.

A good supplement would have natural forms of vitamin E, and all of its varieties. Natural vitamin E has "mixed tocopherols and tocotrienols." In addition, they should be the "D" version (e.g., "d-gamma-tocopherol"). Synthetic and less active versions start with "DL" instead of "D."

Check their whey protein and quality.
A good quality whey protein comes from pesticide and chemical free grass fed cows. Protein manufacturers who use these quality ingredients will make sure you know about it from their packaging and information labels. It is best if these proteins also are cold processed and filtered so the proteins are not damaged, and the whey keeps its full immune system boosting elements. These kinds of whey products are least likely to cause allergies and most absorbable and beneficial.

Yes, it does take a bit of work to find supplements that are well made but think of it this way … a company that will, by choice (because there is no law) make the best possible product even though it means it cannot compete on price, is probably a company that cares about you.

9.8.3 The hierarchy of supplements

Without asking you to take too many lab tests, I will divide the most common nutrient deficiencies that I have found via laboratory testing with my clients and the results that I have seen. This should give you a good idea of what supplements would help you get a better outcome without taking an excessive number of pills.

Note: It is more important to take note of the nutrition guidelines given in **(Chapter 9)** before starting to take the Tier 3 or lower supplements. Supplements are exactly that, additions to an already sound nutrition plan. They cannot overcome a bad lifestyle by themselves.

The best illustration I have heard about the usefulness of supplements is that they are like a stylish tie while a good lifestyle and nutrition plan is like a finely crafted shirt. You will already be well dressed wearing just that shirt alone but a nice tie can add more style. However, it would be foolish and weird to wear a tie without a shirt no matter how wonderful the tie is.

Tier 1 supplements

- Digestive aids—It doesn't make sense to spend time and money on supplements if you are unable to absorb them. That is why the first tier of supplements includes those that support your digestion **(Chapter 4)**. This usually means some kind of HCL supplement at least for most people.
- Methylation support—If you have the MTFHR gene. Methylation is one of the detoxification pathways in your liver **(Chapter 11) but** some people, mostly Caucasians have a gene that makes the process inefficient, increasing disease risk and slowing metabolism. They require a high dose of "methyl donors." The way to find out if you have this gene is if you have smelly urine after eating asparagus.

Tier 2 supplements

The nutrients that I have found commonly to be deficient in many clients fall into this tier. Adding them is very likely to help you.

- **Omega-3**—The benefits of omega-3 are literally too many to count. They benefit every section in this book and in your body, from sleep, to brain function to exercise results and more.
- **Magnesium**—Magnesium is possibly the supplement that gives the most immediate, noticeable benefits to the most number of clients because it helps them sleep better within one or two days. It also is involved in more than three-hundred known reactions in the body and helps everything from stress management to premenstrual syndrome symptoms, to fat burning. Vitamin D and E also are required for magnesium absorption, so if supplementation does not seem to have an effect, check these two other vitamins also.
- **Zinc**—Zinc also is a nutrient that is involved everywhere. It is especially deficient in people who consume or have consumed

large amounts of alcohol, and in those who are under a lot of stress. Lack of zinc slows down metabolism, digestion and sex hormone production. The zinc taste test **(4.2)** can show you if you need some.

- **A good multivitamin**—This should aid detoxification and cover most baseline nutrient needs
- **Vitamin D**—Sorely lacking and beneficial to everyone in some way or another because vitamin D receptors are found on EVERY cell in your body. Especially useful for places where the sun does not shine for many months each year. Although even in equatorial cities, most people spend the sunny hours of the day indoors. The darker your skin color, the more you will need.

Tier 3 supplements

These supplements are used when you need a specific benefit from them, have an increased risk factor or when a lab test shows that you are functionally deficient.

- **Vitamin C**—Is needed to make serotonin a relaxing brain chemical **(Chapter 6)**. It also is a powerful antioxidant and is depleted by stress.
- **B complex**—boosts energy and metabolism of food, improves relaxation, depleted by stress. You can add additional B-5 (pantothenic acid) if you are under high stress as they help protect your adrenals (stress glands).
- **Vitamin E**—Improves insulin resistance and reduces the bad effects of high blood sugar (glycation). An excellent antioxidant, especially so for the female reproductive system.
- **GLA**—A good kind of omega-6 fat that boosts metabolism and is useful for premenstrual syndrome symptoms and balancing our fat profiles in your body.
- **Carnitine**—Necessary for fat metabolism. Move to Tier 2 if little/no red meat is consumed or you are a vegetarian.

- **Reduced "R" form alpha lipoic acid**—Helps manage blood sugar and protects your liver. Slows aging probably by reducing oxidative stress as it recycles other antioxidants like vitamin C, E and glutathione.
- **Resveretrol**—Anti-aging, heart protective, brain protective and cancer protective benefits are well as boosting insulin sensitivity **(9.9)**.
- **CoQ10**—Helps produce energy in cells, very important for heart conditions. This is almost always deficient in people who have a history of taking cholesterol lowering drugs.
- **Green tea**—boosts metabolism for up to twenty-four hours and has high antioxidant properties in its polyphenols.

9.9 Insulin sensitivity

When trying to burn fat and use energy efficiently, one of the key things that we try to accomplish is to improve insulin sensitivity of our cells. When your cells are insulin sensitive, every time you eat, you are more likely to send nutrients to your healthy muscles and organs, rather than storing it as fat.

A good way to think about this is what I call the "gym owner" analogy. Imagine that you and your competitor have each opened a gym. Both of you have equally good training equipment, both gyms are equally well taken care of and maintained, both gyms have equally well educated coaching staff. In short, they are equal in almost every way… except one…

The price of parking for clients of the gym. Your gym represents a fat cell, and your competitor's gym represents a muscle cell. In our bodies, muscle cells have expensive parking, and fat cells have free parking (i.e., muscle cells are naturally less insulin sensitive than fat cells, and nutrients tend to get stored in fat cells rather than muscle cells).

In the gym owner analogy, your gym (muscle cell) has very expensive parking, and your competitor's gym (fat cell) has very cheap parking. This means that all other things being equal, you will tend to store fat rather than build and replenish muscle.

This is the "normal" state of things in most people's bodies, and everything we do with training, nutrition and supplementation is aimed at making your muscle cells more insulin sensitive and their parking cheaper so nutrients tend to go there rather than into fat cells.

9.9.1 How does one make him/herself more insulin sensitive?

Here are some simple actions that all of us can do to boost insulin sensitivity and reduce insulin resistance:

- Do strength training—it boosts insulin sensitivity, which long slow cardio does not.
- Consume healthy fats, in particular omega-3s and mono-unsaturates from sources like olive oil.
- Cut our refined carbohydrates. For obese people, I would limit this to only non-starchy fruits and unlimited vegetables.
- Sleep well, as sleep deprivation makes you more insulin resistant.
- Manage stress levels. Do some relaxing stuff daily (e.g., writing a journal, hanging around with positive people, and smiling are some simple things that everyone can do).
- Take nutrients that boost insulin sensitivity and help blood sugar issues.

9.10 Common Nutrition Questions

9.10.1 Is too much protein bad for my kidneys?

This is one of the oldest and most unfounded myths ever. The reality is, that there is no evidence either research-based, or in practice, that shows that protein damages kidneys, except in one case—pre-existing kidney conditions. If a person already has failing kidneys, then yes, they should not be taking in excess protein. However, what is the likely cause of kidney damage? Actually, excess refined carbohydrates cause it!

So, unless you have a damaged kidney, protein from high quality sources is fine. Think of it this way… Is running up stairs a good form of exercise that will help to keep you healthy? Yes, it certainly is a good form of exercise. However, if you have a pre-existing injury on your legs, then no, running up stairs is no longer a good exercise for you.

9.10.2 How important is vitamin D?
Simply put, it's extremely important. Vitamin D has receptors on every single cell on your body. Therefore, it certainly has a multitude of important functions. It's long list of benefits are just starting to be discovered but here are some well-known ones:

- better immune system health to prevent annoyances like the flu,
- fewer allergies and autoimmune diseases because vitamin D helps to make sure your own immune system does not attack your body with "friendly fire,"
- fat burning because it helps your thyroid to boost your metabolism,
- reduced risk of diabetes because of better blood sugar management,
- reduced risk of most cancers because vitamin D presses the "self-destruct" button of cancer cells called "tumor necrosis factor alpha," and
- muscle building because vitamin D improves testosterone levels naturally.

The best way to get vitamin D is by exposing yourself to sunlight. Even the best quality supplemental vitamin D is not as good as the vitamin D produced in our own bodies when we are exposed to sunlight.

In fact, Dr. Michael Hollick, probably the world's number one expert on vitamin D, has researched and found out that vitamin D produced from skin exposure to sunlight lasts longer (two times or more) in our blood as when it is taken as a supplement because more of the co-factors for vitamin D production are made when we make it ourselves.

9.10.3 Isn't too much sun bad for us?
The risk-to-benefit ratio of having sunlight versus not having it is excellent.

The most common damaging problem of excessive sun exposure is what is known as basal cell carcinoma, a form of skin cancer. Certainly, it is not a good idea to get skin cancer.

However, basal cell carcinoma is relatively non-malignant, and almost never results in death. However, the cancers that have a lower risk with higher sun exposure (we know this because they are more common in less sunny areas of the world) are very deadly. Colon, breast, prostate and others are very dangerous cancers and the factors against them are all influenced positively by sunlight and good vitamin D levels.

I don't mean to be "morbid" but we all probably know many people who have passed away from cancer. However, how many of them had skin cancer? Hardly any. However, many of them had the deadly versions of cancer listed above.

However, we need to condition ourselves to sunlight and our bodies will adapt.

Sunlight has two types of ultraviolet rays (UV), Type A (UVA) and Type B (UVB). UVB burns us but also stimulates vitamin D production. UVA tans us but also is damaging to the skin. Most sunscreen blocks only UVB. So, we don't get vitamin D production. Yet it allows us to feel "unburnt" so we stay longer in the sun, and absorb a lot of UVA, which eventually causes skin problems.

In short, if we are not accustomed to sun, we will be burnt, that is the sign that we have had enough and should go inside. However, sunscreen "turns off" the burning and helps us stay outside longer than our current tolerance allows.

It is a bit like exercise. If a person is conditioned gradually (getting a tan over time) he can withstand great physical training and stress. However, taking a suntan lotion is like training while on painkillers, you feel no pain so you don't know when to stop and you get a serious injury because your body actually cannot handle the sudden increase in exercise load.

So how much sun should we actually get for maximum vitamin D with minimum risk? Dr. Hollick gives some guidelines that my clients and I have followed with great success. I will use equator sun as the benchmark, along with a person who has moderately tanned skin.

For a person like that, twenty minutes, in a singlet and shorts three times a week in the midday sun would be a good starting point. Don't ever get burnt. If you get any shade of pink, that is probably a bit much already.

If you have very fair skin, you need less time and if you have dark skin, you need more. If you move to a country further from the equator with different seasons, you will also need more.

Some practical tips include eating lunch outdoors with your sleeves rolled up, participating in outdoor leisure activity during your off days and weekends. Check your levels with a 25(OH)D test **(Chapter 9)**. If this amount is insufficient to raise your vitamin D levels, take a good vitamin D3 supplement in a relatively high dose of 5,000 to 10,000 IU per day, and re-test in a few months to see where your levels are now. A good amount is about 8ng/mol, which is higher than most laboratory norms but then again, most lab norms are for the average person, who is not in great health.

9.10.4 What are the best ways to cut out carb cravings?

Have you wondered why it's so easy for some people to stick to healthy food habits, while others yo-yo between different diet gurus, diet books and diet ideas, never getting any long-term results?

I have had people starting out at Genesis Gym saying how it has been hard for them to stay away from certain foods because they are "addicted" to those foods.

The new member simply can't even bear the thought of changing their lifestyle. It causes them stress even to consider changing habits, even though they know that trans-fat-laden, potato chips are not good for them.

Why is this the case? Why does it happen to some people more than others? Is it just a case of poor self-discipline?

Here is why food can be addictive and three things you can do about it. Foods produced today are simply too yummy. It is in the big food companies' interest for us to eat more. The way to do this is to make the food super yummy!

Willing buyer, willing seller right? Yes ... kind of but the buyer bears the health consequences, while the sellers get rich.

Wheat products (bread, pasta, all grains) are a major offender, along with sweet things like ice cream and cola. The "most yummy" combination is sugar together with fats and all the bad stuff is basically those two put together:

- chips—starch (sugar) and oil (fat);
- cakes—sugar, flour and oil (fat); and
- burgers—bread (it's the same as sugar to your body) and melted cheese (fat);

and so on…

These processed, yummy foods also tend to be cheap, available, cause negative consequences to your hormones and cell function and are overly dense in terms of energy.

They also have a high "opiate" response in your brain. So, you literally do become addicted. If you stop them suddenly, you can have a mild form of the depression and mood swings that can also be observed in drug addicts who decide to quit cold turkey.

So, we shouldn't get judgmental on people who are fat. It's not only an issue of simple "poor self-control." Let's work on fixing the problem and here are some things you can do.

1. **Manage stress using methods other than food.**

   Carbohydrates can help lower stress levels; that is why students with final exams or people with deadlines tend to eat more starchy food. However, this is a temporary fix. Once the "sugar rush" wears off, you are still stuck facing the stressful event. Just that now you are facing it as a fatter version of your old self!

   Different people use different techniques but here are some that I like.

   - Exercise—too much research on this, just go out and be physically active.
   - Writing a journal—write with a positive attitude and it has been proven by research to reduce stress levels because writing clarifies your thoughts and puts your brain into "problem solving mode" rather than "stressed and whiny mode." I suggest thankful, grateful, positive writing, in addition to lists of things you have learned, how you have helped someone or how you are planning for the future.
   - Mood management natural nutrients—Omega-3 and magnesium are great choices.

2. **Out of sight, out of mind, out of mouth!**

   Several factors encourage overeating (see end of article for research credits):

- food left within reach,
- food left easily visible, and
- bigger spoons, bowls, cups, etcetera.

No kidding.

So keep bad foods—far away in the highest cabinet, out of visible line of sight and if you do eat them, eat with small utensils! Sitting in front of the television with a two-liter tub of ice cream and a large spoon is a bad idea.

3. **Chose foods that make you full.**

   Foods that rate highly on the "satiety index" of how full they make you feel tend to keep you away from the cookie jar. These foods tend to have:

   - more fiber,
   - more protein,
   - more water, and
   - slow absorption/digestion.

   Nuts, meats, low glycemic index fruits such as oranges and apples and berries, leafy veggies and beans tend to score well. Candy bars and doughnuts do not! In addition, a quick tip I have used is a tablespoon of heavy cream plus five grams of the amino acid glutamine. It really shuts down carb cravings!

9.10.5 Are preserved foods okay?

Some people say preserved and canned food is excellent for convenience, while others say it's a major health risk. So what do you need to know about these kinds of food that can help you maximize your health? Let's start with some things about the items contained in preserved foods. Some of the common methods used to preserve food are:

- **Drying**—This is a fairly good method of preserving food. It usually doesn't add artificial ingredients. The one thing you need to know is that it can cause you to eat "more" and that can lead to unwanted fat gaining.

For example, dried grapes (raisins) or apricots are a lot smaller than their "full-sized" fresh versions. You can end up eating a lot more of them. This can lead to a shocking amount of excess sugar and calories. So beware of that.

- **Freezing**—This also is a good method. In fact, most studies show that frozen foods keep almost all of the nutrient content of fresh foods. Most vitamins (e.g., A, D, E), most fiber and all minerals are not affected by freezing.
- **Nitrates**—These are usually found as sodium nitrates especially used in meats and fish. This can cause the formation of nitrosamines, which have been linked to increased risk of cancer. So keep these to a minimum.
- **Salt and sugar**—If the food has these as preservatives it is best to rinse these off. Draining off the excess sugar or salt solution, followed by a nice rinse off can about halve the salt or sugar content of the foods. You can also choose a low salt/sugar option.

Note: Many cans use Bisphenol-A linings that are known to be disruptors of your hormonal system (specifically the reproductive hormones!). So, to avoid this. Try to get things from glass bottles if possible.

So, what are the recommendations I give my clients?

- Choose wisely and try to get stuff in glass containers.
- Drain and rinse foods stored in salt or sugar.
- It's still good to eat canned/preserved foods. Eating a can of preserved veggies or meat is better than giving an excuse about how you can't find some healthy foods and ended up eating potato chips instead.

In a case like this, you may not be able to get the "best option" of freshly prepared, nutritious food but you are still able to find the least bad solution, even if it comes in a bottle or can.

9.10.6 Why can't I just exercise after eating all of the bad food I like?

One of the common misconceptions of new clients at Genesis Gym is that they can "burn off" a bad meal by doing some exercise after. This is an idea driven by the negative emotion of guilt. I will explain why this method of guilt-based exercise doesn't work, and how to plan a "less healthy" meal into your week.

First, let's take what I call the "pizza" example.

Let's say you go to a party the night before and overdo the pizza eating. According to Domino's website, half a regular peperoni pizza (four slices) is 1160 calories. This has 135g of carbohydrates and 51g of fat. Then guilt kicks in and you decide to go for a jog. "That will burn it off" you think. So, you take a 100-minute jog, which is way more than normal but the thought of that pizza sticking on your love handles helps you push through the sore knees to finish the jog. "Phew, I got rid of those 1160 calories!" you might think. Not so fast... Here is why this method will not work.

1. **Food is not just calories. Food is information (9.1)** telling your body what to do.
   In this case, the large amount of carbohydrates in the pizza stimulates the storage hormone insulin, and gets stored in your fat cells. The large amount of fat in the pizza, combined with insulin also get stored in your fat cells.
2. **We tend to eat bad food at night.**
   The high fat levels lower growth hormone output, which is a critical part of the fat burning and body repair processes that we need to do at night.

3. **The exercise we did with good intentions quite possibly did burn 1160 calories.**

However, it is a long, slow, cardiovascular dominant form of exercise, which when done for long periods of time (needed to get rid of ALL of those calories) tends to:

- break down muscle for fuel since amino acids are an important fuel for long activity;
- raise stress hormones, which means fat storage especially around the tummy area and even further break down muscles for fuel; and
- lead to an overall lower metabolism and easier future fat gain because of the increased fat and lowered lean muscle.

As you can see the "burn off a bad meal" mentality doesn't work well.

So what shall we do?

- Normal daily food should be unprocessed and "caveman" in nature **(Chapter 9)**.
- If you do eat a bad meal, try to make it more carbohydrate-based with limited amounts of fats together with it. Eat it several hours before you sleep.
- Use strength training as your main form of exercise. It builds lean mass and this increases insulin sensitivity of your muscles, which means that nutrients from meals will tend to replenish your muscle stores rather than get shuttled into your fat cells.
- If you do go overboard, don't worry. It can happen to anyone. Just recover quickly and get back on track. Be more particular about your food choices and quantities **(9.6.3, 9.6.4)** for the next few days.

9.10.7 Why can't I just count calories?

The "advice" given to overweight people by most health care providers is to eat less, count your calories and eat below your maintenance requirements.

This method has many flaws, including difficult adherence, lowered metabolism, loss of lean muscle and possible nutritional deficiencies if you care more about cutting calories than you do about eating enough nutritious food. Most glaring of all is that it doesn't work for many people.

Despite the restrictive lifestyle they put themselves on, they don't seem to get much result. This is backed by research showing that the effectiveness of a calorie restricted diet plan was VERY dependent on the current state of the individual person. The main difference in question was what is known as insulin resistance.

Simply put, a person who is insulin resistant tends to put any nutrients eaten into their fat stores (i.e. they get fatter). A person who is insulin sensitive (the opposite of resistant) tends to put their nutrients into muscles and organs for use and to be burned off.

For people who are insulin sensitive, all kinds of diets worked well for them (e.g., high carbohydrate, high fat, low fat, balanced plans). So, they are the lucky ones. With a high carbohydrate diet they dropped about nine pounds and with a low carbohydrate, high fat diet they dropped 11.7 pounds.

For the people who are insulin resistant, the results of the low carbohydrate, high fat diet were far more effective. With a high carb diet, they dropped only 3.3 pounds, and with a low carbohydrate diet, they dropped 11.9 pounds.

So, no matter who you are, a low carbohydrate, high healthy fat (e.g., coconut butter, animal fat, nuts, avocados) diet will work and if you are insulin sensitive, almost any diet will work. Aside from helping you reduce weight, being insulin sensitive also reduces cardiac and diabetes risk, and tends to allow more stable energy levels throughout the day **(9.9.1)**.

9.10.8 Don't I need milk for bone health?

One of the fallacies that is often spread is that calcium is the sole key to bone health, especially for women and especially as they age. Supplement and dairy producers have made millions on this assumption.

While calcium is an important mineral, many factors can affect its effectiveness, and how much calcium you eat is just one of them.

You can take in all the milk or calcium supplements in the world but if the rest of the system is not in balance, it won't help your bone strength much. In fact, with the questionable quality of processed milk in most places, along with lactose intolerance being a common problem, especially among people of Asian descent. I prefer to get calcium from other sources like leafy vegetables (e.g., spinach, kale), beans and seafood.

First, you want to avoid loss of calcium. One major factor in calcium loss from bone is excessive acidity. This comes in many forms, usually from carbonated drinks (it's the phosphoric acid!), excessive exercise and stress.

So sleep well **(Chapter 3)**, remove sodas and perform resistance training (which has a net bone strengthening effect) rather than excessively long cardio sessions.

The next thing to do is to make sure that you are getting enough calcium and that it is well absorbed. The co-factors (stuff that calcium needs to work with) that are most important are Vitamin D and magnesium.

Vitamin D is available easily through sunlight and vitamin D is explained here **(9.4.2)**. Magnesium is hard to get from food because of lower soil and food production quality and that is where I usually suggest a good magnesium supplement **(9.8)**.

To ensure good absorption, you will need a good digestive system. Making sure that you have good levels of digestive acid and good bacteria in your digestive tract are critical **(Chapter 3)**.

For this, probiotics and a good amount of unprocessed foods in your diet is a good idea. As you can see, excessive dumping of calcium and poor absorption of calcium can be caused and fixed by multiple factors, which all work in a web of causes and effects.

Unfortunately, there isn't a single bone health solution despite what some companies would like you to believe. That is just the way our wonderfully complex body works. Just get the basic ideas right and you will probably never have to worry about bone health.

Chapter 10

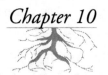

LABORATORY TESTING

S imon was one of our hardest working clients and committed to good nutrition and training but he was unable to drop those last few pounds around his waist and belly. Despite some nutritional changes the belly fat remained. After a month of trying different training and nutrition strategies, I recommended that he take a food allergy test along with a comprehensive metabolic profile.

From the test results, we found that he was intolerant of some "healthy" foods including sea bass, broccoli and celery. In addition, he had a functional deficiency in several critical amino acids and B vitamins.

Once we took out the foods of which he was intolerant and used higher doses of these nutrients to supplement his already healthy diet, he dropped 3.8% of body fat within six weeks without eating less or training more and finally was able to see his abdominal muscles for the first time in his life.

Key Point: Laboratory testing is a time saving solution if consistent, healthy habits are in place, yet results are not coming.

This chapter will cover the main lab tests available in the market to help determined the cause of more difficult health conditions. It will cover the best labs to use, and the most commonly used tests.

It's best to do these tests through a well-informed doctor. It is my personal belief that practitioners shouldn't overcharge for these tests apart from administration fees or the fee for drawing your blood. You can check around for the prices in your country to make sure you are getting a decent deal. The way health care practitioners do add value and should be chargeable is the consultation and follow-up that they can provide you once the test results are in.

10.1 Common laboratory test information

The most common general health check that you will get as part of a regular checkup or corporate health plan usually consists of the following:

- height, weight and BMI—not a good indicator of what's going on unless you are very overweight. See section **(2.3)**;
- blood pressure—good overall indicator. A good number is 110/70. However, make sure it is measured correctly **(5.5.6)**;
- EKG for your heart—not that useful unless it is a "stress EKG" because it is possible to have a heart attack with a "normal" EKG reading. The stress EKG is the one done with you on a treadmill;
- cholesterol checks—incomplete picture **(4.5.5)**
- HS-CRP—a good indicator of overall inflammation.
- Triglycerides—a good indicator of overall excess recent carbohydrate intake;
- blood sugar—too easily affected by recent food intake; and

- hemoglobin A1C—a good indicator of overall glycation **(9.3.3)**, which is an indicator of excess carbohydrate intake over the last three months.

These can give you some indicators of health and is useful, especially blood pressure, stress EKG, HS-CRP, triglycerides and HA1c.

10.2 Other laboratory tests
Unfortunately, because of the complexity of each person the varied genetics we have and environments in which we have lived, I have had many clients who come in with good overall health checkups but still have issues with their weight, sleep, digesting, energy levels and/or brain function. If the previous chapters have not been able to help you overcome those problems, a more comprehensive lab test can give you clues that you can look into for further improvements.

Just like everything else in the world, there are varying qualities of labs. I will recommend labs that both my clients and my colleagues in medicine around the world have found to be accurate. There are many books that can be written about lab testing but I will be providing the most common tests I have used and how they can help you.

10.3 Food intolerance tests
The number one lab test that I would run if I were facing a client who did not have good results so far, is a food intolerance test. The reason is that foods that are healthy in general but not well handled by your particular body can be a big obstacle in your path to a happy body.

They can increase inflammation, stress hormones, digestive tract problems, brain related illness, fat storage and cause all-around havoc! It is hard to sleep well, burn fat or feel good under these conditions. The good news is that once the offending foods are taken away, you can get a significant improvement within days.

The best food intolerance test by far, is the mediator release test by Signet Diagnostics. This is the most accurate food intolerance test around because it tests for inflammation rather than simply your body's immune response to a food, which can give too many false positives according to what you have eaten a lot of recently.

The only downside to this test is that it is only available in Europe and North America, because of the need for a fresh blood sample within twenty-four hours. Only Europe and the USA have labs and even the best courier service can't get the blood to the lab within that time from further away.

The next best option is the "ALCAT test" or the "Metametrix Labs IgG4 serum antibodies" test. These require a medical professional to draw a small blood sample for you. If such a person is not available easily, you can use a test you can do by yourself. For self-testing, my colleagues and I have found the "Food Detective" home testing kit works well and while it may not test the widest variety of foods, it does gives you a good result within an hour or so, which is far quicker than waiting two to three weeks for the lab results to come back.

10.4 Comprehensive metabolic profile.

The second test that has worked really well is called the "Comprehensive Metabolic Profile" (CMP) from Metametrix Labs. This test covers the basic version (thirty versus ninety foods) IgG4 food intolerance test, which uses a blood spot (so, no need for a nurse or doctor to draw blood), as well as what is known as an Organix profile and an amino acid profile. These three tests together are called the CMP, or TRIAD profile.

10.5 Organic acid test

The Organix profile is an organic acid test (OAT), which checks your urine. These acids are the intermediate products of biochemical processes. For example, if there is a process in your body that produces substance B from substance A and we find too much of A, then we know that there is trouble turning A into B and can focus on a solution to this "blockage." This block can be caused by a lack of nutrients, lack of enzymes for this pathway, a toxicity problem or even a bacterial overgrowth.

As listed on the Memetetrix Lab website, this test is a good way to find out if you have:

- vitamin and mineral insufficiencies;
- amino acid insufficiencies like carnitine and N-acetyl cysteine (NAC);
- oxidative damage and antioxidant sufficiency markers;
- indicators to assess detoxification sufficiency;
- the best functional markers of B-complex deficiency;
- neurotransmitter metabolites to assess central nervous system (CNS) function;
- mitochondrial energy production assessment via citric acid cycle components;
- methylation sufficiency status;
- lipoic acid and CoQ10 sufficiency markers; and
- specific dysbiosis markers for bacterial and yeast overgrowth.

The results of the test are returned to you in a PDF file and give very detailed descriptions of the findings for your body, the problems this finding causes and some nutrient and lifestyle changes that can help you overcome these problems.

Here is an example of the information you may get from the organic acid test... As you may have read in **(Chapter 12)**, I am not a fan of large amounts of aerobic exercise for health or weight loss. Sometimes clients may disagree with me until we show them the results of their OAT. There is actually part of the OAT, which checks for one of the damaging effects of excessive cardiovascular training. High levels of oxidative stress **(Chapter 7)**.

This test is called "8-Hydroxy-2'-deoxyguanosine" or (8-OHdG). Don't worry about the super nerdy name. This compound is a by-product of oxidative damage to DNA and it can be measured in urine. Of all the clients in our gym who have taken this test, only two had elevated levels of 8-OHdG. These two were the ones training for endurance activities like marathons and triathlons. In fact, their levels were way off the charts (more than eleven units when acceptable range is less than 5.3, and ideal is somewhere around two or three). This shows us that, if you are an endurance athlete, it is best for you get huge quantities of a variety of antioxidants like vitamin C, E, selenium, glutathione, alpha-lipoic acid and stuff from brightly colored fruits and veggies **(Chapter 9)**. This is just one of the dozens of markers that the OAT can give you, which you can use for maximum health.

10.6 Amino acid profile

This test also is part of the CMP and will give you a summary of how your body is handling amino acids, which are found in every single tissue in your body. The test checks for all the amino acids that affect:

- cardiovascular function,
- brain neurotransmitters,
- detoxification and antioxidant function, and
- ratios between types of amino acids.

From these results, you can add in the nutrients that you lack and perhaps cut back on those of which you have excess.

10.7 Fatty acid profile

Another test that can be added to the CMP is the Metametrix fatty acid profile. I like to use this with clients who may have eaten large amounts of processed foods and bad oils in their past. It is a finger prick, DIY blood test and can be done at the same time as the CMP.

From the Metametrix website, this test can show the following information:

- Inflammatory balance. Improper fatty acid intake affects the balance of anti- and pro-inflammatory eicosanoids, increasing health risks.
- Statins. Among the top five drugs prescribed last year, statins have been shown to alter this inflammatory balance unfavorably.
- Increased free radical production. Consumption of polyunsaturated fatty acids (PUFAs) without increasing antioxidant intake will cause increased production of free radicals.
- Immune suppression. Excessive consumption of omega-3 fatty acids can suppress immune function, leading to infections and poor wound healing.

10.8 Stool tests for bacteria

If your organic test **(10.5)** shows some bad bacteria issues in your digestive tract, it is best to do a full stool analysis to see what's going on. Metametrix has a test called GI effects, and Doctors Data Lab has a test called the "comprehensive stool analysis."

10.9 Heavy metals

In general, there are three kinds of tests for heavy metals:

- live blood cells,
- urine, and
- hair.

While they all have their uses, the most useful one probably is hair. Apart from Dr. Schauss **(10.11)**, the other leading expert on heavy metal toxicity who's work I would suggest you read if you suspect that heavy metals are an issue, is Dr. Andrew Hall Cutler.

10.10 Genomic testing

Genetics only give tendencies and certainly don't determine your fate because your genes can express themselves very differently depending on your environment, diet and lifestyle, which are under your control (9.7, 5.4.2). However, you can get an idea of these tendencies along with potential gene mutations.

For example, if you find out that you cannot detoxify diesel fumes well, it's best not to get a job in the petrochemical industry. Alternatively, if you find out that you have a risk for heart disease and you find that you have low amounts of heart protective omega-3 (10.7), you would certainly be motivated to add some into your diet.

For genomic testing, "Genova Diagnostics" has excellent tests for different risks including detox, breast cancer and heart conditions, "Fitgenes" in Australia, and "23 And Me" are more general but also give good information.

10.11 What if this is not enough information?

As you consult with your doctor and learn more about lab testing you will find that each lab has many options for testing. If you are still not sure, I suggest you find the number one man in the world (in my opinion) whom you can contact to get a consultation. He is my mentor in lab testing, Dr. Mark Schauss.

His book, "Victory Over A Toxic World" is a must have for those who are serious about their health. Dr. Schauss writes from the perspective of both a scientist, as well as the father of a child suffering from seizures about which no one else seems to have a clue. So, that sets him upon his journey of learning about lab testing with great passion, skill and enthusiasm.

Because of his wide range of experiences in the "health industry" while finding help for his daughter, I believe he has a very balanced viewpoint about both the pharmaceutical as well as the alternative fields of health care. His points are made in (nice!) short chapters so you could probably pick up this book and read it from any point instead of front to back. He also has an excellent, free, podcast on issues related to health research and lab testing. It is called "Let's Talk Real Health". It can be somewhat technical at times because he is explaining a complex topic, but if you are interested in more information in this field, it is a wonderful resource.

Chapter 11

DETOXIFICATION

Phyllis is one of the fittest women at our gym. She can perform chin-ups and can squat 75kg for five repetitions when she weighs just over 50kg. These are good performances for almost any woman athlete. Since she joined, she also dropped her body fat from 28% to 19%. However, despite a healthy lifestyle and good training, she still stored most of her fat on her lower body around the buttocks and hips, while having a lean upper body. A fat storage patter like this is usually a sign of high levels of un-detoxified, excess female hormones.

One of the best ways to handle this kind of problem is a detox. Phyllis did seven days of a detox program designed to give her body the nutrients and environment that boost her estrogen detoxification pathways. The detox included high levels of nutritious medicinal foods, organic vegetables and a lot of estrogen clearing nutrients like Di-indoly-methane, and fiber to clear the estrogen via her stool.

One week later, she had dropped almost one centimeter of fat on her buttocks, and after her second week, she had dropped almost two.

Key Point: A targeted detox can help you break through a plateau or overcome a health condition.

This chapter will cover how increased toxicity affects our bodies. This is an area we need to be more and more aware of as our surrounding environment is more filled with thousands of chemicals, pesticides and hormones that were not around even a hundred years ago. There will also be a short explanation of how our body reacts to toxicity and how we can support our body's natural detoxification ability.

11.1 What is toxicity?

Toxins can take many forms. They can include things like cigarette smoke, petro-chemical fumes, plastics, pesticides, microorganisms, heavy metals and excess or unwanted hormones like sex hormones, and stress hormones. When you are exposed to toxins of any kind, your body does it's best to reduce their impact. They get stored in a progressive manner. From my experience, one of the best models that explains how this happens is by Dr. Hans Heinrich Reckeweg. It is expressed in this six-stage model below.

Stage 1 In this model, the body starts with healthy detoxification systems and a low amount of toxicity. In this case, the toxins are cleared out well. This happens through several different routes **(11.2)**.

Stage 2 As the level of toxicity goes up, there is inflammation and this activates the body's immune system. From this activation, you may get symptoms such as allergies, acne, coughing, frequent illness and other infections.

Stage 3 If toxic load increases further, your body has no choice but to store the toxins and it tries to store them in the "least bad" location. It tries to protect your cell function by storing the toxins in the space outside your cells. Once you get to this stage, there are symptoms such as chronic allergies, bladder/kidney stones or gout.

Stage 4 If toxic load increases further, things start to get really bad, because this is when the toxins start to get into your cells. The symptoms from the previous stage tend to die down but rather are replaced by a general feeling of fatigue. Chronic diseases such as arthritis, heart failure, chronic infection and chronic gastritis are signs of this stage.

Stage 5 If toxic load increases further, the cell loses its ability to perform its functions. The symptoms are serious problems such as chronic fatigue, liver cirrhosis, diabetes, multiple sclerosis and **amyotrophic lateral sclerosis (ALS).**

Stage 6 In the final stage, under a toxic load that is high and un-detoxified, the cells no longer function and no longer even look like the cells they are supposed to be. To protect the rest of your body from the highly toxic, damaged cell, the damaged cell "hides" itself in a shell—this is a tumor. In fact, 86% of biopsies of cancer cells have found some kind of toxin in these cells.

As you get deeper into the stages of toxicity, another effect on your body is a slower metabolism. Your body does this as a protective mechanism to reduce the impact that toxins have on it. Many of the cell's functions are dependent on electrical activity at the cell wall passing things in and out of the cell. This means that there needs to be a difference in electrical potential between the inside and the outside of the cell. Just like you need a slope (a difference in height or gravitational potential) to push things up and down a hill.

It is estimated that approximately one third of a cell's energy is used to maintain this electrical potential. When a cell is toxic, it is not able to produce this energy and the potential drops, often leading to a lower metabolism and likely weight gain.

11.2 How does my body detoxify?

Our bodies need to clean out an estimated five-hundred or more different toxins per day. Toxins are mainly stored in fat-soluble forms but your body can only eliminate toxins in four ways. Through your stool, your urine, your sweat and your breath, all of which are water-based. It is the function of your liver to convert these fat-soluble toxins into water-soluble forms for elimination.

It does this in two phases, both of which are very dependent on nutrients. In Phase 1, some toxins are neutralized but others are "activated" into forms that are then neutralized by Phase 2 nutrients.

For proper function of Phase 1, here are some of the critical nutrients:

- B vitamins,
- folic acid,
- glutathione,
- antioxidants,
- branch chain amino acids,
- carotenoids,
- vitamin E,
- vitamin C,
- vitamin A,
- N-acetyl cysteine,
- quercetin, and
- calcium.

For Phase 2, here are some of the required nutrients:

- selenium,
- sulphur-based molecules (usually from cuciferous vegetables),
- carnitine,
- N-acetyl cysteine,

- amino acids such as:
  - » glutamine,
  - » glycine,
  - » taurine,
  - » cystine, and
  - » arginine.

At each of these phases there are free radicals produced. So, you need to have enough antioxidants **(5.5.2)** to protect yourself from these free radicals. Without the right nutrients listed above, you are far more likely to have a poor detoxification system and that leads to toxin accumulation that progresses further and further **(11.1)**.

While it is true that there is a wide variance in each person's ability to detoxify different toxins, anyone who adds poor nutrition, excess alcohol and high levels of stress to the list of problems, will find that their detox processes go much slower and toxins are more likely to build up.

Once the toxins are converted into water-soluble forms, they can be excreted by stool, urine, sweat and breath, generally in that order. If a person has exceptionally smelly sweat, or breath, that's a sign that there is insufficient capacity to excrete toxins via stool. They need to check their digestive tract health **(3.1)**.

11.3 What should I do to detoxify well?

Note: Try to be aware of which stage of the six-stage model you are in **(11.1)**. If you are at Stage 4 or worse it is best not to do a detox unsupervised. Consult an experienced medical practitioner. It can take a lot of time to detox safely from that point on because when there is a lot of toxic load; detoxification is a great stress and burden on your body and needs to be managed well.

If you are within Stage 1 to 3, and have no history of other health conditions, you can probably do a detox that will be successful by following the guidelines below. The guidelines work best as a lifestyle not a "one off" solution. After all, if you are following the guidelines in each chapter of this book, you will accomplish most of the detox guidelines given below and should have a good overall detox ability. However, with the current levels of toxicity in the world, it is helpful to perform a full week of healthy detox once or twice per year.

Detox guidelines

- "Turn off the tap" **(1.1)** gets away from this source of toxins. Parabens, pythlates, petrochemicals, plastics, solvents and estrogens are common toxins. The excellent website EWG. org has a great resource for finding out where common and uncommon sources of toxins are.
- Do not follow a fruit juice or soup-based detox program. They simply don't provide enough nutrients for a good detox.
- Make sure your digestive tract works well. Fix any gut conditions **(4.2)**.
- Make sure you have the right amount of nutrients for Phase 1 and Phase 2 processes **(11.2)**.
- Make sure Phase 1 and Phase 2 are going at a balanced rate. This means taking in enough nutrients for both phases. Most "juice detoxes" only focus on Phase 1 nutrients, which over burdens Phase 2 and leaves you feeling worse than before in the long-term.
- Make sure you have the right amount of antioxidants required to clean up the mess that detoxification causes.
- Make your energy production system (Kreb's cycle) work.

Points three to six are very nutrient dependent. If you need them and don't supply them (not enough in your food) or don't absorb them (poor digestive health), you will cannibalize them from your body's current stores. This means you will usually break down lean muscle tissue as well as bones. Following the hydration and nutrition recommendations in **(Chapter 9)** is a good place to start. However, the following supplements can aid you greatly especially if you know you are a slow detoxifier or have been in a location or job that is more exposed to toxins. They are listed in order of what I have found to work well, and this is a good starting point. However, each individual may have different priorities, which can be found via lab testing **(Chapter 9)**.

- a good multivitamin **(9.8.2)**,
- digestive aids listed in **(4.2)**,
- magnesium,
- vitamin D,
- omega 3,
- methylation support especially if you have smelly urine after eating asparagus,
- electrolytes, and
- amino acids especially if you do not eat much animal protein.

11.4 How do I do a one-week detox?

The basics of this cleanse are taught by renowned nutritionist Dr. Robert Rakowski who is my "go to" guy for all kinds of nutritional questions, especially for clients who may have challenging health conditions. This also is the cleanse that helped Phyllis (the story at the start of this chapter) get over some of her hormonal imbalances and fat loss plateaus.

This is a very basic version of the cleanse. However, it will still do wonders for almost everyone. If you have a long history of illness or fatigue or are a high-level athlete, it is best to consult with a functional medical practitioner, and perform some lab testing **(Chapter 9)** to see what else you may need to add to the detox plan for maximum results. However, this is still a good basic plan to start with.

1. Select the medicinal foods for your condition. If in doubt, choose an inflammation reducing food, and an estrogen detoxifying food.

2. Choose one kind of organic veggie per day (e.g., day one—spinach, day two—asparagus, day three—green beans).

Eat UNLIMITED amounts of the medicinal foods and veggies for seven days.

3. Do some physical activity each day, at least a brisk walk and ideally some resistance training. **(Chapter 12)**. This causes lymph fluid to flow and boosts immune system activity.

After the seven days, take two scoops of the medicinal food each day, add in three to five grams of omega three supplements, and if you don't eat much veggies, add in one tablespoon of a greens supplement.

4. Stay clear of all common allergenic "problem" foods by following a modified elimination diet. This is the plan that I give to clients whom I suspect have a food intolerance problem.

Modified Elimination Diet – Food Choices		
	To Select	To Avoid
Fruits	Unsweetened fresh, frozen, water packed, canned.	Oranges
Veggies	All fresh, raw, steamed, sautéed, juiced, or roasted	Corn, creamed veggies
Starches	Rice, oats, millet, quinoa, amaranth, tapioca, sweet potatoes	Wheat, corn, barley, spelt, kamut, rye, all products containing gluten

Cereals/ Breads	Products made from rice, oats, buckwheat, millet, potato flour, tapioca, arrowroot, amaranth, quinoa	Products made from wheat, spelt, kamut, rye, barley, all gluten containing products
Legumes	All beans, peas and lentils	Soy beans, tofu, tempeh, soy milk, other soy products
Nuts/Seeds	Almonds, cashews, walnuts, sesame (tahini), sunflower and pumpkin seeds, butters made from these nuts and seeds	Peanuts, peanut butter
Meat & Fish	All canned water packed, frozen or fresh fish, chicken, turkey, wild game, lamb	Beef, pork, cold cuts, sausages, canned meats with preservatives, eggs, shellfish
Diary	Milk substitutes like almond, oat, coconut and outer nut milks	Milk, cheeses, yoghurt, cream, ice cream,, non diary creamers
Fats	Cold pressed olive, flax, sunflower, sesame, nut based oils, pumpkin oil	Margarine, butter, processed oils, mayonnaise, spreads
Drinks	Filtered or distilled water, herbal tea, mineral water	Soda and soft drinks, alcohol, coffee, tea, other caffeinated drinks (energy drinks etc)

Spices	All spices e.g. cinnamon, cumin, dill, garlic, ginger, carob, oregano, parsley, rosemary, tarragon, thyme, turmeric, vinegar etc	Chocolate, ketchup, mustard, chutney, soy sauce, BBQ sauce, other pre-made, and processed sauces
Sweeteners	Brown rice syrup, fruit sweetener, blackstrap molasses, stevia	White and brown refined sugar, honey, maple syrup, corn syrup, high fructose corn syrup, candy, desserts made with these sweeteners

11.5 Detoxing specific problems

As an extension of section (11.2), there can be specific problems related to genetic tendencies (some people just clear out certain toxins better than others), as well as your environment.

For example, one of our clients' jobs was to inspect the safety of the storage tanks of oil tankers. He did so for years without protective equipment or breathing apparatus because it is hot and stuffy in there. As might be expected, he needed support to detoxify petrochemicals before he got good results from his fitness program.

Here are some common toxins, their sources and the nutrients and habits that will aid their detoxification. As might be expected, rule number one is always REMOVE yourself from the source of the toxin (12.1).

Plastics

One of our clients was a researcher in a local university. His job was to research plastics for aircraft parts. He had his head in a fume cabinet for many hours per day creating these plastics. The plastic-based toxins he absorbed affected his energy levels, sleep quality and ability to burn fat. As expected, he needed some detox for plastic before he started to get better results. Plastics also are known as a cancer-causing toxin; so, it's best to clear them out as much as you can.

Other, perhaps less obvious plastics sources can be:

- eating utensils and containers,
- water bottles,
- dentures,
- non-stick coating on cookware,
- paint, and
- plastic products of all kinds (especially those with softer plastics).

Far-Infrared Sauna

If you suspect that plastics may be an issue for you, the most effective way to remove plastics, in addition to the basics of detox in **(10.3)**, is by using a far-infrared sauna. We use this in our gym with great results. After all, most of us live in big cities where plastics are very common. Make sure to take some amino acids and a wide spectrum antioxidant like a greens drink, as well as some reduced form alpha-lipoic acid about twenty minutes before entering the sauna. These supplements will support your liver during the sauna session.

Sauna sessions should start short and at your own personal level of tolerance. The detox may cause some mild headaches or a lightheaded feeling from the toxins. Come out if this happens. Fifteen minutes or so is a good starting point. Make sure to bring in a towel and keep wiping yourself off to prevent toxins re-absorbing into your skin. Shower immediately after.

One interesting observation is to keep your sweaty towel in a plastic bag on your way home. When you open the bag, check out the smell. If toxins came out (which is usually the case) the towel will smell a lot worse than just sweat. From my experience, when a toxic person does the sauna, his towel smells more like garbage than sweat. It may also have a grey residue on it.

Estrogens

As explained in the section on cancer **(5.4)**, excess estrogens are a serious problem. Nutrients that are well known to boost the ability of your body to clear out estrogens are:

- diindolemethant (DIM),
- sulphorophane,
- calcium D-glucorate,
- curcumin,
- flax hulls,
- probiotics (also SB), and
- resveratrol.

In addition, you can support the liver in Phase 2 by making sure you have enough B vitamins and folic acid. The amino acids cysteine and taurine also are beneficial.

Petrochemicals

The most useful pathway in the liver for clearing of petroleum-based toxins is glycination. As such, the amino acid glycine is an excellent choice if you have been exposed to high levels of petrochemicals or feel particularly unwell, for example, at a gas station.

The way to take glycine is to start with a small dose of about one gram (one fifth of a teaspoon) taken with your last meal of the day. Increase this dose by one gram each day until the next day gives you loose stools. This is a sign of overly fast detoxification and from that amount, you can back off a gram or two for the optimal current dose for you.

Heavy metals

Heavy metal issues can be complex and should be detoxified under the care of an experienced functional medical professional. However, the lab tests **(Chapter 10)** for heavy metals can give you an indication of whether you should be looking for a doctor to help you.

Some safe things that you can do yourself if you suspect heavy metal issues are:

- bentonite clay and modified citrus pectin to help bind heavy metals in your digestive tract,
- far-infrared sauna, and
- soaps that can clean up heavy metal particles. A good example is "D-lead" soap from Esca Tech.

Chapter 12

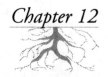

EXERCISE

Note: All exercise programs are demonstrated on the book's website. It is very hard to teach with just words and pictures. And it is also hard to show the effort level required for great results unless you see it in action.

D oreen is actually my mom! At age fifty-eight, she is what I would consider a role model for healthy aging. How does she do it? Very importantly, she has a great attitude towards people, work and life, helping many people in need, formerly as a volunteer for the Samaritans of Singapore, a non-profit call hotline for people in need, as well as part of her duties as a church elder. This willingness to give of herself helps to keep her stress levels low.

She also eats unprocessed food almost all of the time, along with basic supplements such as omega-3 and a multivitamin. Finally, she stays STRONG and still does deadlifts and squats at my gym. Most impressively, she is able to do three chin-ups (yes, man-style chin-ups).

Main point: Getting old is guaranteed but aging is optional.

Admittedly, exercise for health is a pretty new idea. The idea of doing MORE physical activity was not common because for most of human history we had to do a lot of physical work simply to survive. Either walking long distances to forage, sprinting to hunt animals or working the fields for hours per day in subsistence farming. Any extra, free time was spent resting!

Today, with super busy schedules, many modern conveniences and sedentary jobs, most people do need to dedicate some scheduled time for physical activity. I will be describing exercise as used for health reasons in this book. Specialized training for high-level athletes is certainly one of my favorite areas of study but they are not directly relevant for most readers.

The main goals of most people's exercise program should be to burn fat and to build lean muscle. They work in combination with the nutrition guidelines of Chapter 8 to accomplish this result. So, what kinds of exercise should you be doing? For how long? Do you need equipment? In this book, I will present the principles that my team and I have used to help thousands of people over the years in our training centers.

12.1 Your schedule?

In an ideal world, we would all have plenty of time for exercise. If a client had a totally free and flexible schedule, two short but hard training sessions per day would be ideal for best results. As you can imagine, for people with a job, social and family commitments training two times per day is rarely an option. In fact, often it is not the perfect training program but the one that a client can do within their schedule limitations, which is the ideal one for them.

In all of our initial consultations, I try to negotiate for four sessions of physical activity per week as a minimum. They don't all have to be hard sessions, especially for people who haven't trained for a while but training often (not necessarily long) has shown in practice and in research, to give better results. The reasons for this are not yet clear but it does seem to be the "way we are created" to be active daily. So the closer we get to daily activity, the better. Four to five short sessions seem to give more results than one or two very long ones.

Because time is limited, it is important to get the most benefits out of each minute you dedicate to exercise. There is a psychological component to training and you are more likely to do the training that you enjoy. All activity is probably good for you but you need to dedicate your time to activities that maximize your results per hour. This is because you don't have unlimited time to exercise unless you are a professional athlete.

If you have less than three hours per week to exercise.
In my experience, this is the majority of general population clients that we see. If this is your situation, your main activity should be strength training. It gives the biggest "bang" for your "buck" in terms of benefits per minute of training time.

If you have between three to five hours per week.
You can add in some interval training by playing sports, by riding a bike or working on a stair climber, rowing machine or on a running track.

If you have more than five hours per week to exercise (quite rare).
You can add in some relaxing cardio sessions. I suggest a nice relaxing walk on the beach or in a park with your family. This is generally a good idea because it is a mild form of exercise that does not add extra burden to your recovery systems and stress glands and probably helps you distress. So, you can do as many of these as you like.

The program in this book will give options for all people with differing schedules.

12.2 What kind of exercise?

12.2.1 Aerobic Training—A.K.A "cardio"

The most common form of exercise that people take up is some form of cardio. The benefit of this is that it is easy to pick up and can be done almost anytime, anywhere.

The problem with cardio-based training is that it doesn't work well for fat burning or muscle building, the two most important aspects of a training program for most people. In fact, in exercise physiology studies since the 1970s, cardiovascular exercise has been shown to serve almost no advantage in fat burning over simply changing your nutrition as shown in (**Chapter 9**).

For example (there are many), a study in April of 2011 took a group of 399 obese and sedentary women. They were divided into three groups:

- one group did exercise alone,
- one group did diet changes alone, and
- one group did both exercise and diet.

The exercise chosen was cardio for forty-five minutes, five times per week. This is quite a lot of exercise, certainly more than most people do. This added up to almost two-hundred hours over the course of the twelve-month study.

In the end, the group that did both diet and aerobic exercise dropped only 1.8kg (four pounds) extra fat compared to the group that did diet changes only. This is quite a waste of two-hundred hours! In addition, excessive cardio has other drawbacks including:

- increased stress hormones,
- decreases in hormones that maintain lean muscle,
- increased inflammation and oxidative stress, and
- lower immune system function.

All of these negative effects make sense considering the fact that long cardio sessions appear to the body as if you are lost in the jungle or in a prisoner of war camp. That is stressful and the correct thing for your body to do is to store fat just in case you don't have enough to eat. This is undesirable in our age of excessive food availability in most developed countries. Simply put, working up a good sweat on a treadmill or elliptical trainer doesn't mean much when it comes to actually burning fat. You may lose weight, but unfortunately, much of that is likely to be your precious lean muscle tissue.

12.2.2 Strength training and interval training

The two beneficial alternatives are strength training and interval training. When a strength program is well designed, it can give you the benefits of interval training as well, all in one training session. That is why a person who is pressed for time will do best on a strength-training-based program. The program outlined in this book is based on strength training.

Note: The exception to this rule is a person with a pre-existing cardiovascular condition. If you have very elevated blood pressure or a heart condition such as valve or heart chamber issues, you should work with a well-qualified medical professional and trainer for best and safest results. In general, if you have these conditions you will need to work on your cardiovascular capacity with some longer, slower exercise first, generally progressing to faster cardio then to strength training once you are well adapted to training. This is one of the few times that a focus on cardiovascular based exercise is the best option.

12.2.3 Benefits of strength training, in contrast to excess aerobic training, strength training, when planned properly, has a multitude of benefits including:

- increased lean mass,
- improved immune system function,

- increased insulin sensitivity,
- increased metabolism,
- increased flexibility,
- decreased risk of injury,
- fast recovery if you do get an injury, and
- looking healthy lean and strong!

It is these multiple benefits with minimal negative effects that should encourage you to spend the majority of your available training time on resistance training if you are looking for the best results.

12.3 Training programs

There is no "perfect" exercise program. That being said, there are some principles that will make the programs in this section well suited for a majority of people, both male and female.

You will find this book will have two training programs that should last you about eight to twelve weeks of training. These programs are excellent ways to start developing good technique and habits in a gym. I will only use dumbbells and a bench in these workouts because that is what almost every gym has.

If you have no gym access, I will explain how to set up an affordable home gym. If even that is not possible, then you will still be able to exercise using basic equipment, along with your body weight. Complete training videos will be available at the happy body website.

Principles of these training programs:

- They will be based on resistance training because it gives you the most benefit per minute of exercise.
- They will train your entire body because this gives the greatest overall release of fat burning hormones.
- They will alternate exercises between upper and lower body because it demands that your body shifts blood around more, increasing caloric expenditure.

- They will have sets that last about forty to seventy seconds because that is the kind of set that helps you build lean muscle.

You will have 'incomplete' rest between exercises. This kind of structure gives you a greater "burning" feeling that further stimulates fat burning hormone release.

12.3.1 How to read a training program
The programs in this book are read from left to right.

There is a lot of information in a program because how you perform a program determines the benefits you receive. All of the parameters here are geared to help you gain lean tissue and burn fat.

First column
- The first column is the order in which the exercises are to be done. Do "A" before "B" and B" before "C" and so on.
- The numbers after the alphabet indicate that these exercises are to be done is a circuit fashion. If you see A1 and A2, it means do a set of A1 followed by a set of A2, then A1 again then A2 again.

Second column
- The second column is the exercise name. There will be pictures in the book, and videos online with coaching tips for each exercise.

Third and fourth column
- The third column is the number of sets of each exercise and the fourth column is how many repetitions you should aim to perform. One set is all of the repetitions done before moving to the next exercise. For example, if you see three sets with ten to twelve repetitions, it means you should do the exercise ten to twelve times using a resistance that is challenging (you

couldn't have done thirteen repetitions!) but not too heavy (you can do at least ten). This may take some guesswork to figure out the first time you train.

Fifth column

- This number is the tempo of the exercise. It indicates how fast or slow you should do the lifts. There are four numbers in this column. For example, "4-0-2-0." The first number is how long (in seconds) it should take you to lower the weight. The second number is how long you should pause at the bottom of the lift, the third number is how fast you should lift the weight, and the final number is how long you should pause at the top of the lift.

Sixth column

- This number is the length in seconds that you should rest before moving on to the next exercise.

12.3.2 Warming up

Before you start exercise, you should do the warm-ups that suit the activity you are about to perform. For strength training workouts, we will stretch the parts that are often tight in people who have sedentary jobs. Following that, we will do a warm-up set of the exercises in the workout. That should be enough warm-up for most people, without taking up too much training time.

Warm-up activity:

- foam roller relaxation if time permits,
- hip flexor stretch,
- hamstrings stretch,
- calves stretch,
- pectoral stretch, and
- latisimus dorsi stretch.

Descriptions for these stretches above are found in (7.4).

These are just the most common areas of tightness that we have found in sedentary clients. Flexibility and methods for increasing it can take up a series of books on their own. If you have difficulties with flexibility, the best book on this subject is called *Stretch to Win* by Ann and Chris Frederick. Alternatively, you can seek out a qualified fascial stretch therapist in your area.

12.3.3 Training program one

Day One

Order	Exercise	Sets	Reps	Tempo	Rest
A1	Front Foot Elevated Split Squat	4	10-12/side	3-0-3-0	60
A2	One Arm Row To Tummy	4	10-12/side	3-0-3-0	60
B1	Dumbbell Stiff Leg Deadlift	4	12-15	2-0-2-0	45
B2	Neutral Grip Incline Bench Press	4	12-15	2-0-2-0	45
C1	One Arm Trap Three Raise	3	8-10	3-0-1-2	30
C2	Front Bridge	3	Hold 60 sec	Hold 60 sec	10

Day Two

Order	Exercise	Sets	Reps	Tempo	Rest
A1	Heel Elevated DB Hack Squat	4	10-12/side	3-0-3-0	60

A2	One Arm Row To Neck	4	10-12/side	3-0-3-0	60
B1	Front Step Up On Heels	4	12-15	2-0-2-0	45
B2	Standing One Arm Shoulder Press	4	12-15	2-0-2-0	45
C1	Standing External Rotation Arm At Side	3	8-10	4-0-1-1	30
C2	Side Bridge	3	Hold 30 sec /side	Hold 30 sec /side	10

12.3.4 Training program two

Note: Do this after four to six weeks doing program one

This program uses what are called "extended sets" which use changes in the exercise to keep you pushing deeper into fatigue to give a greater lean muscle building, and fat burning stimulus for your body. On the exercises with just ten seconds of rest, that means simply move quickly to the next exercise and begin.

Day One (Upper body)

Order	Exercise	Sets	Reps	Tempo	Rest
A1	Supported Row To Tummy	4	6-8	4-0-1-0	10
A2	Supported Rows To Chest Pronated	4	12-15	2-0-1-1	180
B1	Incline, Neutral Dumbbell Press	4	6-8	4-0-1-0	10
B2	Decline Pronated Dumbbell Press	4	12-15	2-0-1-1	180

Day Two (Lower body)

Order	Exercise	Sets	Reps	Tempo	Rest
A1	Forward Lunge	4	6-8/side	4-0-1-0	10
A2	Heel Elevated Dumbbell Squat	4	12-15/side	3-0-1-0	180
B1	Side Step Up On Heels	4	6-8	4-0-1-0	10
B2	Dumbbell Romanian Deadlift	4	12-15	3-0-1-0	180

Day Three (Shoulders and arms)

Order	Exercise	Sets	Reps	Tempo	Rest
A1	Neutral Seated Unsupported Dumbbell Shoulder Press	4	6-8	4-0-1-0	10
A2	Lying Dumbbell Triceps Extension	4	12-15	2-0-1-1	180
B1	Seated Hammer Curl	4	6-8	4-0-1-0	10
B2	Incline Curl	4	12-15	2-0-1-1	180

Progression

Getting better is an important part of training. If you haven't trained in a while, start with "half" a workout. Simply do half the number of sets that are called for. If the program says four, sets, do two, and if it says three, do one or two. Each time you try out the program try to increase either the repetitions by at least one or the resistance by 2-5% from the previous time you attempted that same workout.

12.3.5 Interval training program

To get started with interval training without worrying too much about measuring distances or worrying about which machine or method to use, I like to use what is called the "perceived exertion" (PE) scale.

Simply put this is a scale from one to ten with "one" being the effort you would be exerting, and the difficulty you would get from a slow stroll on the beach with your family and friends. A "ten" would be the exertion and effort you would be feeling if you were being chased by a pack of wild dogs.

Here are two good interval programs. You can use any method you prefer (e.g., rowing, swimming, running, hill sprints, stair climbing, cycling). It is best to switch up your method every few weeks to keep your body from getting used to a method and "too efficient" at it, which produces a lower fat burning effect.

Interval program structure one
- five minute warm-up—PE 3/10
- two minutes fast—PE 8/10
- four minutes slow—PE 3/10
- repeat this fast/slow pattern three to six times depending on fitness level
- five minute cool down—PE 3/10

Interval program structure two
- five minute warm-up—PE 3/10
- thirty second fast—PE 9/10
- three minutes slow—PE 3/10
- repeat this fast/slow pattern four to eight times depending on fitness level
- five minute cool down—PE 3/10

12.3.6 Travel workouts

Because training is actually less important than nutrition, your main priority during your time away from home is to find a place to get nutritious food. When my clients travel, I just ask them to do the interval-training program **(12.3.5)** once per day using different machines.

However, if you do want a basic travel workout here are two options. One is just bodyweight and one is with a simple and fairly affordable device called a TRX. Many brands make similar devices so choose one that fits your budget and has the attachments that suit you. For example, the TRX has a door attachment that can be fixed to any sturdy door.

Bodyweight workout one

Order	Exercise	Sets	Reps	Tempo	Rest
A1	Prisoner Split Squat	4	8/side	4-0-1-0	10
A2	Push Up (kneeling if too hard)	4	12	4-0-1-0	10
A3	Lying Glute Bridge	4	12	2-0-1-2	10
A4	Front Bridge	4	60 sec hold	60 sec hold	10
A5	Birddog	4	8/side	2-0-1-3	120

Bodyweight workout two

Order	Exercise	Sets	Reps	Tempo	Rest
A1	Step Up	4	8/side	2-0-1-0	10
A2	Narrow Push Up (kneeling if too hard)	4	12	4-0-1-0	10
A3	Rear Foot Elevated Split Squat	4	8/side	4-0-1-0	10
A4	Side Bridge	4	30 sec hold	30 sec hold	10
A5	Burpees	4	As many as possible in 60 sec	2-0-1-0	120

TRX Workout 1

Order	Exercise	Sets	Reps	Tempo	Rest
A1	Rear Foot Elevated Split Squat	4	8/side	4-0-1-0	10
A2	Inverted Rows To Tummy Palms Down	4	12	3-0-1-1	10
A3	Hamstring Curls	4	12	3-0-1-1	10
A4	Flat Chest Press	4	12	3-0-1-1	10
A5	Ab Rollouts	4	12	3-0-1-1	120

TRX Workout 2

Order	Exercise	Sets	Reps	Tempo	Rest
A1	Single Leg Squat	4	8/side	4-0-1-0	10
A2	Inverted Rows To Chest Palms Neutral	4	12	3-0-1-1	10
A3	Bicycle Hamstring Curls	4	12/side	2-0-1-0	10
A4	Chest Flies	4	12	2-1-1-1	10
A5	Bicycle Abs	4	12	2-0-1-0	120

12.4 Common questions about exercise

12.4.1 "What about my heart health? Don't I need to do cardio?"

This common question is asked when we show a client their training program. Of course, I am a big believer in having a healthy heart—and who isn't? However, the common misconception is that an hour on the treadmill or stair climber is the best way to give you one.

In reality, you can get a double benefit from well-designed strength training programs because they benefit your heart as well. Cardiovascular training does not have a monopoly on heart benefits. Here is why. The cardiovascular system and heart are not directly "trained" (i.e. you don't stick a mini-gym in your chest and train your heart).

The heart responds to demands of the body. In the case of exercise, the cardiovascular system is responding to the demands of the muscular system. The heart does not care if you're lifting weights, playing basketball or swimming. If the amount of training is sufficient, and the rest periods short enough, your heart does not care if you are playing a game of basketball, swimming, running or lifting weights, your heart will get a positive training effect. So, why not do strength training and get the heart benefits and more.

12.4.2 "Why can't I just eat whether I want then train it off later?"

Check out **(9.10.6)** for the pizza example, and why this won't work.

12.4.3 "What workout should I do if I just ate a heavy, unhealthy meal?"

If you do this consistently, nothing will work for you. However, if you enjoy a big feast occasionally, don't panic. There isn't a magical workout that can burn it off in a healthy way. Just go back to your healthy habits, and cut back on carbohydrate and portion sizes for the next day or two.

12.4.4 "Will strength training make ladies big?

Part of our job as coaches is education. Education leads to better compliance to the program, and thus better results. One of the main areas of education we need to work on with our female clients is to help them overcome the "fear" of having more muscle.

This is a reasonable fear since women have the commonly portrayed image of female bodybuilders and their bulging, steroid fueled physiques running through their minds when they think of lifting weights. What women do get, in fact, is a firm, lean, athletic physique. Any "big arms" are because of bad food choices much more often than too much resistance training. Here are three big reasons it's great for women to do resistance training to build lean muscle.

1. **It makes you more resistant to illness.**
    Resistance training boosts lean muscle mass and bone density and mass. This is great news because bone and muscle are the main stores of the nutrients you need to boost your immune system.

    Also, the nutrient stores in your bone and muscle are where your body turns to in times of excess acidity. This is important, because being more alkaline helps with immunity, stress management, brain function and detoxification.

2. **It makes you leaner.**
    Having more lean muscle boosts metabolism. This is hard to measure but most nutrition experts guess this to be about one-hundred calories per day per kilogram of muscle. Also, resistance training makes your muscles more "insulin sensitive." What this means in simple terms is that nutrients will be attracted into your muscle cells rather than your fat cells, which means less fat and lower blood sugar and diabetes risk. (As a side note, long cardio does not give you this benefit) These two factors make having lean muscle a great benefit for women who want to burn fat.

3. **It makes you live longer.**
    A Tuft's University study found that the amount of lean muscle you have is a far better predictor of long life than cholesterol levels and blood pressure! So, the greater lean mass you keep for life, the more likely that life is going to be long. The second more important factor for long life was closely related. It is

how strong you are. Resistance training also is called strength training because it certainly helps here too.

So women, if you want to stay illness-free, burn fat efficiently, and live healthy and long, resistance training is critical. Ideally, you do four sessions a week of at least forty minutes for best results combined with some form of stretching and light activity like walks with your friends or family.

12.4.5 "Will strength training reduce my flexibility and coordination?"

One of the other reasons that people may have reservations about strength training is that there is an old myth that being strong means you become inflexible, slow or clumsy. This is actually true—in the short run. However, this clumsiness will go away if you keep practicing your sport or activity.

For example, I had a client who was a Ballet and Jazz dancer. She wanted to get stronger so that her dancing movements would be more powerful. This would be perceived by her audience as more graceful. Dance, after all, is a tough activity to train for!

Within a few weeks of starting her training with us, she came up to me and, with some discouragement in her voice said: "I don't think your training plan is good for me, I stumble and fall more than before!" I said: "*Great! It's working!*"

What is happening is that in your muscles there are two kinds of feedback sensors called golgi tendon organs (GTO) and muscle spindle cells. Spindle cells are responsible for feedback of position, and golgi tendon organs feedback tension.

When you train seriously, your muscles change size and your spindle cells are not in the same positions as before. So, the feedback they give to your brain is different and your brain does not receive and in return, does not give the right signals back to your muscles. Also, your GTOs are not used to the new tensions placed on them by the training, their feedback also is new and different, and you stumble and look more clumsy.

This "problem" takes approximately twenty-one days to reset. That is why when we train high-level athletes, we give them an adjustment period before their competitions or performance.

So, the key piece of advice is to use strength training properly! Train really hard until three weeks before your competition or performance, then just maintain your strength and size. This will allow your body to be both strong and coordinate the new strength. So, a combination of understanding anatomy and strength training leads to great results.

Another fear is the strength training makes you "tight" and inflexible. This is actually the opposite of what occurs when training is done correctly with full ranges of motion in the joints. Instead of becoming tighter, your body will actually get more flexible because it will be stronger, and more able to control your joints at their end ranges of motion. This will make the brain think—"Oh, I'm stronger now. It's okay to let my joints go farther without getting injured." Thus, you will be both stronger and more flexible!

Two weeks later my dancer client remarked how much better her flexibility, speed and strength had become. This is exactly what can be expected when we give our body a chance to adapt to its new abilities. So make sure to include some form of strength training with all of its benefits to your exercise plan.

12.4.6 "Should elderly people do strength training?"

It is easy to see that even as medical technology advances we have been able to live longer and longer. That is great news. According to studies by the World Bank, the life expectancy in my country Singapore has gone up from about sixty-six years in 1960, to about eighty-two years in 2009. I believe this is the pattern in most developed countries as well.

However, longer life isn't that great. Who cares if I live to be a hundred-ten years old but can't walk, am in chronic pain, can't take care of myself, and need a machine to help me breathe and go to the toilet? The issue in question is not length of life but rather, quality of life.

If a senior client comes to our training center and wants to know what changes they can make to their life to increase its quality, there is a long list. There are medical tests you can to do check your body's ability to detoxify and digest. There are supplements that can aid your body's ability to recover from stress and there are food plans to help you manage your blood sugar, body fat and weight.

However, if there were just one top lifestyle change to recommend, it would be strength training. Not cardio, not slow walks in the park but a safely designed (according to your current fitness and flexibility level) strength training program. Here are three big reasons why strength training is the right lifestyle habit to learn.

1. **Strength training improves upper body strength and lower body power.**

   How many senior citizens do you know who have come home from a walk to the supermarket, suddenly start panting uncontrollably leading to them being unable to take care of themselves? While this is possible, it doesn't happen often. Cardio vascular conditioning, while important, is not often an immediate factor in quality of life.

   What is far more common is that a person gets older, weaker from lack of activity and then is unable to take care of him/herself. They also have falls because of a lack of lower body strength and power to "catch" themselves if they get off balance for any reason.

   Once a fall occurs, it often comes with a break in a major bone like the hips or legs. This leads to more immobility, less strength and a steady decline in physical ability. This is a terrible decrease in quality of life. Strength training can help with these issues.

2. **Strength training increases cardiovascular and bone health in minimal time.**

   If you had to choose a form of exercise, strength training is your best bet, at any age, and particularly as you get older. When done correctly it boosts cardiovascular function. The heart is not a muscle you can train directly. If you can't make it do pushups, you can't make it go swimming.

   The heart only responds to demands placed on it by the rest of the body. So, if you do strength training in the right way, your heart will get a great workout without wasting time on the bike or treadmill.

   Strength training also boosts bone strength. The healthy stresses placed on the body stimulate bone thickening and strengthening. All of the calcium supplements in the world will not be effective if the body is not stimulated to put it on the bones.

3. **Strength training puts your body into a positive state.**

   You know one of the "secrets" of celebrities looking young is the addition of growth hormone, which can be taken orally or injected. However, the hormonal output of proper strength training programs also is growth hormone! For free! This hormone tells your body to keep and grow lean, strong muscle and bone and it signals your body to drop excess fat. It's "double happiness"!

   Strength training is far more effective at growth hormone release than long, slow cardiovascular exercises. So, it puts your body into a positive hormonal state. Many studies, including one done at the Center of Hip Health and Mobility in Vancouver Canada have found that strength training, which requires more concentration and focus than sitting on a recumbent bike, has the ability to boost brain function. Just two times per week was found to boost memory and decision-making ability in people aged sixty-five to seventy-five years. Loss of memory and brain function is a great fear of many seniors I have spoken to, so keeping your brain in a positive state also is a great increase in quality of life.

Emotional health also is boosted by strength training. Yes, other forms of exercise can get you this benefit as well but it comes "for free" along with the other superior benefits of strength training. The chemicals released from your brain during and after training give an increased sense of happiness, relaxation and wellbeing.

With a good training program, it also is cool to see yourself stronger and fitter than you were thirty or forty years ago! So, strength training boosts confidence as well. All of these factors put your emotions into a positive state.

12.5 Common training mistakes

When trying to achieve a goal, it is often better to focus on what to do right rather than what could go wrong; however, there are usually critical mistakes that you should try to avoid to achieve success faster. In this three-part series, we will discuss ten things that could seriously derail your fitness goals.

12.5.1 Follow a 'magazine' workout program blindly

Unfortunately, many of the workouts in your favorite bodybuilding or fitness magazine are written for bodybuilding professionals, not the average person like you or me. Why does this matter? Well, the people you see in magazines usually have some serious advantages over regular people.

- They are genetically gifted and are naturally quite athletic and fit looking.

- This is their job and they have much more time and energy to train and eat properly than the average stressed Singapore worker.
- They are often on performance-enhancing substances that can have long-term health consequences.

12.5.2 Have no plan

One of the questions my team and I always ask a client when they visit for the first time is, "What is the program you are currently on?" In almost all cases, a random mash-up of exercises and activities may even contradict each other in terms of training goals. For example if you wanted to gain lean muscle while burning fat, long jogs are probably not your best option! Training needs to have a plan because:

- Different activities result in different results. For example, doing heavy weights once or twice makes you strong, and doing light weights many times gives you strength endurance.
- In most cases, if you combine activities wrongly you may get neither of the desired results as your body becomes confused about what to improve.
- If you do not plan and instead train randomly, you cannot track your progress. If this week you focused on heavy weightlifting, next week you decided to do canoeing, and the week after that you decided to do eight-hundred meter runs on a track, it is very hard to determine if you are making progress!
- If you do not plan and train the same all the time, you will stagnate as your body has already adapted to that kind of exercise.

12.5.3 Performing imperfect repetitions

Uncontrolled speed

If you do not control the speed of your exercises, you get different difficulty and training effects. For example, when you do a kipping chin-up (using your legs and body to help you up) you can get better at the skill of doing these kipping chin-ups but you may not actually be getting stronger!

So, to make sure all your repetitions are consistent, make sure that you perform them in a controlled manner. Yes, you will need to lower the weights you use but you will end up with better strength gains. Just give a biceps curl a try with a three-second up and a three-second lowering phase. You will probably get a much better arm workout than you are getting now.

Incomplete repetitions
For most of your training, you should do exercises with a full range of movement. Doing half chin-ups, half squats or half bench presses only develop strength in those "half" ranges. That can lead to muscle imbalances, which increases risk of injury and decrease stability of joints.

12.5.4 Not taking care of injuries when they happen
From the hundreds of consultations my team and I do each year, we can see that most people have had some kind of injury before. Sometimes it is acute or sudden. For example, it is the result of an accident like falling down or a car accident. Sometimes, it is chronic and annoying, such as nagging shoulder, neck or back pain. The keys to handling injuries in an effective way, while not using them as an excuse to get fat and lazy are…

…using the right treatment method for the problem you have

For example, if you were hit by a car, acupuncture is not what you need! You need to go to the emergency room at a hospital.

- For accidents and torn ligaments like your ACL in the knee, a hospital surgery is the way to go.
- For minor strains, acupuncture, massage, soft tissue work and trigenics work well.

- For chronic annoying pain that is bone structure related, a good chiropractor or bonesetter tends to do a good job.
- For chronic annoying pain that is muscle related, the soft tissue massage or the trigenics method works well.
- All injuries do well with good nutritional support. A low inflammatory diet without refined food, along with nutrients like omeaga-3s and curcumin speed healing.

Train "around" the injury

Whenever you have been injured, the best thing to do is to do safe exercises that do not make the injury worse. For example, in my early days, I had a slipped disc injury in my lower back from a sports accident.

It was very painful and I could not lift anything for a few weeks. In fact, even getting out of bed or off the toilet seat hurt. However, two days after the injury I was swimming. I was lifting light weights with exercises that did not involve the back, and as soon as the pain was duller, I started doing light stretches and Mckenzie exercises for my back to help it heal faster. I was back to full strength within a few months.

We never put a person at risk for further damage but training smart and around an injury has the benefit of creating a whole body growth hormone release, which aids healing of your injury even if you are training another part of your body. It also prevents you from getting out of shape. This means you have a shorter road back to full health when the injury is healed.

12.5.5 Not warming up correctly

Most people recognize that warming up before training is a good idea. However, if you read all the articles on the Internet or in books on the subject of warming up, you may come away confused because there are a lot of opinions out there.

Use movement warm-ups or "dynamic" warm-ups for multi-directional or speed activities. For example, skipping, walking lunges, leg swings, are excellent before activities that require changes of direction and speed such as soccer, rugby and sprinting.

Use static stretching for tight parts of your body before all trainings. For example if you are tight in your calves and hips, some contract/ relax stretching (holds of fifteen seconds or more) can be useful **(8.4)**. The increased movement you get will allow you to squat, run or jump with better mechanics, reducing your risk of injury.

Use warm-up weights with the same exercise that you are going to do. For example if I were to do squats in the gym today, and I was trying to lift 100kg ten times, I would warm by squatting with weights up to about 70kg for a few repetitions. During these warm up sets I would use the exact same speed and movement that I would be using for the working sets.

12.5.6 Not progressing correctly

The more conditioned you are to exercise, the harder it will be for you to progress. Our body will not get stronger, fitter or leaner without progress. Progress can come in many ways but it has to be measurable. For example, progress could mean an increase in weight lifted, a reduction in rest time required or an increase in the number of repetitions performed. If you go two workouts without progress, you need to change your program, take more time off or go for a period of lighter training to recover better.

12.5.7 Not changing your workout often enough

There is a kind of fine line to be walked here. On the one hand, if you don't change your training methods often enough, you risk overuse injuries and lack of progress once your body has already adapted to the stimulus of the training. However, if you change your program too often or too randomly, your body has trouble adapting to anything at all.

For example, if you did heavy squats one day, light bench presses the next day, and ran a marathon on the day after that ... your body would be confused about what to get better at. In the end, it is possible that you will hardly get better at any of the three exercises. What a waste of time.

So, in general, you should change workouts after about six of the same workout. This is highly individual but from my experience, it varies from as many as eight workouts for a total new trainee, to as few as one or two workouts for a gifted athlete. Change your workout once you see stalled progress for two sessions. No matter whether your objective is an Olympic medal or to keep yourself healthy as a senior citizen, varying your training program is essential.

Depending on how talented or experienced you are, you will need to change your program somewhere between every two weeks to every six weeks. Unfortunately, most people I see do the same training program for months and even years. The key thing to look out for is lack of progress. In my gym, my staff and I continually monitor client progress and whenever they have two sessions where progress has stalled, the program must be changed because the body has already adapted to the goals that the program has tried to achieve. Doing more of the program has little further benefit and may even increase injury risk.

Two good indicators that you have stalled are: (1) if you are unable to increase the resistance by at least 2% from the previous workout or (2) if you are unable to increase at least one rep from the previous workout.

12.5.8 Changing your workout too often

Yes, this is the complete opposite of what I mentioned in the previous point. However it also is correct. I would guess that more than 95% of people exercising have no plan of what to do.

They go to a gym, get on a bike or go to a track … with no clue what they should be aiming for. As such, they rarely achieve much. In a gym for example, many people go in without a plan and then just end up doing exercises they are comfortable with, are good at or are unoccupied by other gym users. Random training leads to random results. A good guide is to do the same kind of workout for four weeks and then change to a totally different kind of workout for four weeks.

For example, you may focus on fat burning for four weeks where you use circuit training with short rest periods between exercises. Four weeks later, you should switch to a program focused on strength where you use heavier weights and longer rest periods. Four weeks after that, you can focus on a muscle building program with long rests but many exercises for the same muscle group.

The problem with changing workouts too often is that you have no clue if you are progressing because you do totally different things each time you train. As mentioned in point number one, do a workout consistently until you stall, then change it.

12.5.9 Not tracking progress

The saying "you cannot manage what you can't measure" is very true when it comes to exercise. You do need to keep a logbook (just print out the log sheet in the back of the book, or downloadable on the website), to see how you are doing. That's the way you can find out if you need to change programs. Remember, each time you train, you should aim for one more repetition or an additional 2-5% in load.

12.5.10 Using training to overcome bad eating habits

"Oh, right after this meal, I'm going for a run" is one of the things you may have heard or may even have said as you stuffed down the last crumbs of cheesecake from the buffet table.

While I enjoy a good meal just like any of you, it is important to understand that it is next to impossible to out-train bad food habits.

Why?

Even a hard training session uses about six-hundred calories per hour. However, that is just one Big Mac worth of food. Add fries and a soft drink and you are up to more than one-thousand calories. While I'm not a big fan of calorie counting as a lifestyle, it should be pretty clear that it is impossible to eat "whatever I want" and get great results.

The only exceptions to this reality are those who are genetically very adaptable to eating a lot (naturally skinny people who can see their abs and veins even if they don't exercise or eat healthy at all) or those who do massive amounts of activity per day (e.g. manual laborers or professional athletes). However, even this group would still benefit from healthy choices.

So what do you do? You still need to exercise about four hours per week, a decent amount if it is all challenging training. A hard work out in the gym or a set of sprints on the track counts as hard.

Meanwhile, you will still need to make excellent food choices of healthy meats, veggies, good fats like fish and coconut oil and unprocessed carbohydrates like sweet potatoes and some fruit. Also, see **(9.10.6)**.

12.6 What to put in a home gym

Because many people tend to have a hectic an busy schedule, they may choose to exercise at home to save time and stress from traffic jams and packed trains and busses finding their way to a gym.

While a fully equipped gym, along with effort put into performing a proper training program is most likely to get you optimal results, there is a place for in home training when time does not allow you to get to the gym as frequently as you might like.

For clients like this, I am often asked, what to put into a home gym for maximum results. In this section, I will put the items I recommend, in order of priority (and space required!). The prices are approximate and given in 2012 US dollars.

Priority 1—Adjustable dumbbells
Dumbbells are the number one priority in exercise equipment. Despite "cooler" looking and fancier fad equipment that has come out recently, the "old-school" dumbbell, when well used is the most space and cost efficient piece of equipment out there. An adjustable set, which allows you to add weights to suit your current strength, is the best bet. If

possible, get dumbbells that have rotating handles; these are safer for your wrists.

Get plates for the dumbbell in as small increments as you can so you can slowly increase the load as your strength increases. They are made in increments as small as 0.125kg. If these are not available, you can get magnets called "pace weights" that allow small increments too:

- price is $100-$200, and
- space required is 0.5 meters x 0.5 meters.

Priority 2—Adjustable bench

If space allows, the next item to get is an adjustable bench. It should be able to go from flat to about eighty degrees inclined. If possible, get one that goes from about fifteen degrees declined to eighty degrees incline. This will allow a variety of upper body exercises that can be done with you on your back.

Along with the bench, it's a good idea to get something to protect your floor. The mats for children's play areas are a good bet for a home gym and cost about $25 for four pieces of 60cm square:

- bench price is $150-$1500 depending on brand and quality, and
- space required is about 1.5 meters x 1.5 meters.

Priority 3—Squat rack or power rack, along with a barbell

The barbell is another basic piece of equipment that gives more benefits than any fancy gadget available on late night television. To use a barbell to its maximum potential you will need a rack for it. The important thing about choosing a power rack is its hole spacing, ideally, every five centimeters or so. Some poorly designed ones have hole spacing every ten centimeters or more apart. This is not good because we all vary in height, arm-length etcetera, and we need stuff "in-between" to comfortably rack and unrack the bar.

- Rack price: Racks can cost from $150 for a basic squat rack to $4000 for a top of the range power rack.
- Bar price: Bars can cost $100+ to $1500 for home gyms. If you are an average male who wants to train with up to 140kg or so eventually even a cheaper bar will do.
- The more expensive items will last longer but their value is in their calibration, steel quality and warranty. I choose them for our heavy-duty commercial gym use but for home use, choose what fits your budget.
- Space required is about three meters by two meters

Priority 4—Other stuff—Kettlebells, TRX, grip training tools, etcetera

These items are optional extras once the basics are in place. You can add Kettlebells and a TRX before a power rack and barbell but if you had to make a choice, the rack is a better value for your money and space. Because of its portability, the TRX also is an excellent choice for travel workouts. **(11.3.6)**. Finally, get a good training program so you can use this equipment to maximize your results.

Chapter 13

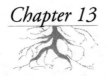

PUTTING TOGETHER
A GREAT WEEK

Let's put all of the things that are covered in this book together to have an excellent week. In this scenario, I will make a few assumptions. In fact, they will be "strict" and many people will actually have a less hectic life than the person I am describing.

Let's take "Jack" as an example for our story. As an engineer in a small manufacturing company, he works regular hours from 8:30am to 6pm. He is of average health. He is slightly overweight at 80kg and 170cm tall and has slowly gained weight while working his way up the ranks to be a senior engineer.

He is 29% fat, most of it stored at his tummy, waist and chest. He exercises by going for a swim at the pool of his condominium once a week during the weekend. Jack's situation is quite typical of the clients I see at my gym.

13.1 A Healthy Day

A good week is made up of good days, but what is Jack's normal day like? Because sleep is so important, let's start from bedtime the day before:

- **12:30am**—After surfing the Internet for relaxation, Jack tries to fall asleep. He lies down on his bed at about 12:30am but usually takes about an hour to fall asleep. He thinks about work, worries about his latest project and what the boss will think of the presentation he just gave.
- **3am**—Wake up and stumble to the toilet to urinate.
- **5:30am**—Jack feels slightly awake but tries to stay asleep because it's not time to wake up yet.
- **7am**—Alarm clock rings and jolts Jack upright in bed. Jack slams the snooze button… "I need just ten more minutes of rest" he thinks…
- **7:15am**—Jack finally gets up out of bed, feeling low on energy and unrested. He brushes his teeth and gets dressed.
- **7:30am** (even later if Jack was a woman and had to decide what to wear, and put on makeup)—Jack goes to the kitchen and makes breakfast: two slices of bread with jam, a glass of fruit juice and a cup of coffee with milk and sugar.
- **8am**—Jack is out of the house and goes to work.
- **8:30am**—Jack arrives at work but still doesn't feel fully focused yet. He grabs a coffee from the office pantry and sits down at his desk. He chats with his colleagues and surfs the Internet for some of today's news.
- **10am**—Jack finally feels focused enough to get down to work. He works for a while but is hungry, so grabs some cookies for a snack—along with another coffee.

- **12pm**—Lunch time, Jack usually eats at the nearest food court, rice or potatoes with two veggie dishes and a serving of meat is his usual lunch. Sometimes it's noodles, sushi or a sandwich.
- **3pm**—The post-lunch, afternoon sleepy period kicks in and Jack dozes off. Time for a cookies and coffee snack.
- **4pm**—Jack is in a semi-dazed state when he gives his presentation. However, the adrenaline kicks in and he survives his boss' tough questions.
- **6pm**—Jack leaves the office, and thinks about going for a swim at his pool but his colleagues convince him to eat dinner with them instead.
- **7pm**—Jack has pasta with some garlic bread and washes it down with a beer.
- **9pm**—Jack watches television and eats a bag of potato chips while doing so.
- **11pm**—Jack finishes his television program and goes online to chat with his Facebook and MSN buddies.
- **12:30am**—REPEAT

Here is what I would tell him… Aside from the fact that he is headed for some serious health issues down the road! Here is Jack "Version 2.0"…

Starting from before bed:

- Make sure his room is dark, cool and quiet. If it's not dark enough, get an eyeshade. If it's noisy, get earplugs and turn on the fan or air conditioner.
- All electronics are off except a battery-operated alarm clock, no Wi-Fi, no hand phone, no laptop, etcetera.
- Thirty minutes before bed he should use a relaxing nutrient combination like glycine and magnesium, which relax the nervous system and your muscles for a restful sleep.

- I would also try to get to bed earlier. The sooner the better because your body rests best from 11pm to about 5am.
- Once Jack starts to get a restful sleep, he should wake up without an alarm clock! That is a sudden, stressful start to the day. Already, he has a stressful job, which causes him to lose sleep because of excess stress hormones.
- More tips and suggestions on sleep can be found in **(Chapter 3)**.
- Once Jack wakes up, I would ask him to eat a nutritious breakfast of meat (yes meat) and a handful of nuts. Why? Meat and nuts are energizing and boost the brain chemicals, which improve concentration, and memory **(Chapter 6)**.
- If Jack defrosted his meat the night before, pan-frying it in butter or coconut oil would take only five to eight minutes depending on what meat he is eating. Zinc and an omega-3 supplement would be a good choice at this time because they help with energy and brain function **(Chapter 9.8)**.
- Jack's current breakfast of bread, jam and sugared coffee is extremely high in refined carbohydrates and will lead to poor morning energy and hunger pangs **(Chapter 9.6.3)**.
- Meat, nuts and healthy fats will give Jack a great, focused, productive morning. I always tell clients to ask their bosses for a raise because their increased health leads to increased productivity **(9.6.3)**!
- At work, Jack will feel ready to work from 8:30am instead of 10:30am. He gets ahead in promotions and bonuses not by working longer but by being more efficient.
- At morning snack time, Jack knows that the cookies and coffee were killing his energy. Instead, he takes some nuts and some carrot sticks he brought from home. This low GI snack digests slowly, and does not give the energy ups and downs that sugary food does. Jack can still have coffee but without milk and sugar **(9.6.3)**.

- Instead, he adds cinnamon powder and heavy cream, which make the coffee digest slower (fewer jitters and energy ups and downs) and actually act as a mild fat burner.
- At lunch, Jack eats something that is nutritious and slow to digest. He eats an herbal soup with watercress and pork ribs, as well as a chicken steak from the western food stall. He swaps the fries for an extra serving of cucumbers and tomatoes.
- Three times a week Jack brings food from home for lunch. He spends his lunch exercising for forty minutes with some interval training at the gym near his office **(12.3.4)**.
- For an afternoon snack, Jack eats another bunch of nuts and carrot sticks.
- Jack has a great presentation to his boss because he is fully able to focus to answer all the tough questions posed to him
- Jack also finds friends who will not sabotage his fitness plans by getting him to eat fattening food like pasta and bread, instead of exercising.
- Instead, he finds friends, family, colleagues, a group exercise class or a coach who will encourage him to exercise. Ideally, four times per week **(12.1)**.
- *"You are the average of the five people you spend the most time with"* I tell my clients. If all of your friends drink beer and eat pizza, you will be fat and weak for sure.
- Jack goes home, plays with his kids and spends time with his wife.
- He also writes a short journal entry with three things he is thankful for today. This reduces his mental stress, and makes him a more pleasant, relaxed and fun dad and husband **(3.3)**.
- Jack limits his time to thirty minutes on Facebook, takes his relaxing nutrients and gets ready for bed at 10:30pm.
- REPEAT

Is Jack 2.0 a superman training for the Olympics? No. He is a person who is serious about maximizing his productivity, happiness and health. He takes good advice and puts it into practice. All people who have exceptional health have habits like this as well.

13.2 A healthy week

- Sunday: Prepare food for the week (one hour), relaxing light physical activity and stretching (e.g., walking, swimming or recreational sports) (one hour)
- Monday: forty-five minutes resistance training
- Tuesday: forty-five minutes resistance training
- Wednesday: stretching
- Thursday: thirty minutes interval training
- Fri: forty-five minutes resistance training
- Sat: stretching

A schedule like that is about right to achieve and maintain great health. To begin, you can do twenty minutes of resistance training instead of forty-five minutes (do only half of a training program from **Chapter 12** for example), and ten minutes of interval training instead of thirty minutes. Slowly build up over a few weeks.

There we have it! It is my hope, that as you read through this book, your appreciation of how wonderfully made and intricately connected your body is has grown. I also hope you have started to gain a greater understanding of how everything from thoughts and emotions, to environment and sleep can either add, or subtract from your overall health. But most importantly, I hope that there is something you have learned, that you can take action on, and do today which will lead to a long term benefits for you and your loved ones' health.

To Your Happy Body,
Coach Jonathan Wong

About The Author

Jonathan Wong is the Master Trainer at Genesis Gym Singapore. He has 12 years of disciplined study and practice in the fields of exercise, nutrition and preventive health care. He developed an interest in exercise and healthcare as a formerly fat kid who wanted to find the best ways to stay in shape. Jonathan holds certifications in varied fields including Functional Medicine, Bio-Medical Acupuncture, Trigenincs, Strength & Conditioning and Personal Training. He is currently studying for his Doctorate of Science in Holistic Medicine and a diploma in Clinical Nutrition.

References

Because this book is so interconnected, it is hard to place certain references within certain chapters. So here is one single list. I will do my best to give credit as much as I can to the work of my teachers, authors and mentors who have helped me in my growth as a coach and health professional. The best thing about learning from them is that they have a combined hundreds of thousands of hours of experience of what works, and what does not. And just as importantly that they are connected to other experts in the field who also get great outcomes for clients and patients.

If I have left any acknowledgements out, please accept my sincere apologies. Please contact me via the book's website www. happybodybook.com, and I will be sure to acknowledge you in future editions, and with an update on the website.

Coach Charles Poliquin
Seminars
- Biosignature levels 1 and 2
- The Poliquin International Certification Program Levels 1 to 4

- Specific training for specific populations – The Stressed Executive
- Specific training for specific populations – Females, with Francine Savard

Books:
- German Body Composition
- Website: www.charlespoliquin.com

Dr Mark Houston
Seminar:
- Cardiovascular health - Nov 2009

Books:
- What Your Doctor May Not Tell You About Hypertension (2003)
- What Your Doctor May Not Tell You About Heart Disease (2012)

Dr Rob Rakowski
Seminar:
- Nutrition & Detoxification – Nov 2009
- Cancer and Natural Treatment - 2012

Dr Johnny Bowden
Books:
- The 150 Healthiest Foods On Earth
- Living Low Carb
- The Most Effective Natural Cures On Earth

Website: www.johnnybowden.com

Dr John Berardi
Website: www.precisionnutrition.com

Dr Alan Austin
Founder of Trigenics
Website: www.trigenics.com

Dr Mark Scappiticci
Designer of the FAT tool, and my teacher in bio-medical acupuncture

Nick Liatsos, Physical Therapist
My mentor in using the Frequency Specific Micro-current device
Seminar:
- Accelerated healing of lower back injuries

Esther Blum
Book:
- Eat, Drink and Be Gorgeous

Website: www.livinggorgeous.com

Dr. Mark Schauss
My mentor in lab testing and detoxification
Seminar:
- Detoxification – Apr 2012

Book:
- Achieving victory over a toxic world

Website: www.toxicworldbook.com

Dr Andrew Hall Cutler

Seminar:

- Mercury Detoxification – Apr 2012

Dr Ann McCombs

Seminar:

- Detoxification & Health – Apr 2012

Dr Eric C. Westman

Book:

- A New Atkins For A New You

Dr. Ron Grisanti & Dr Wayne Sodano

Some of the best functional medicine information and certification available

www.functionalmedicineuniversity.com

Coach Ian King

Seminar:

- Coaching Seminar – Aug 2012

Books:

- Get Buffed
- Winning & Losing

Website: www.kingsports.com

CPSIA information can be obtained at www.ICGtesting.com
Printed in the USA
LVOW12s1952060314

376328LV00004B/320/P